COOKING FOR A
FAST METABOLISM

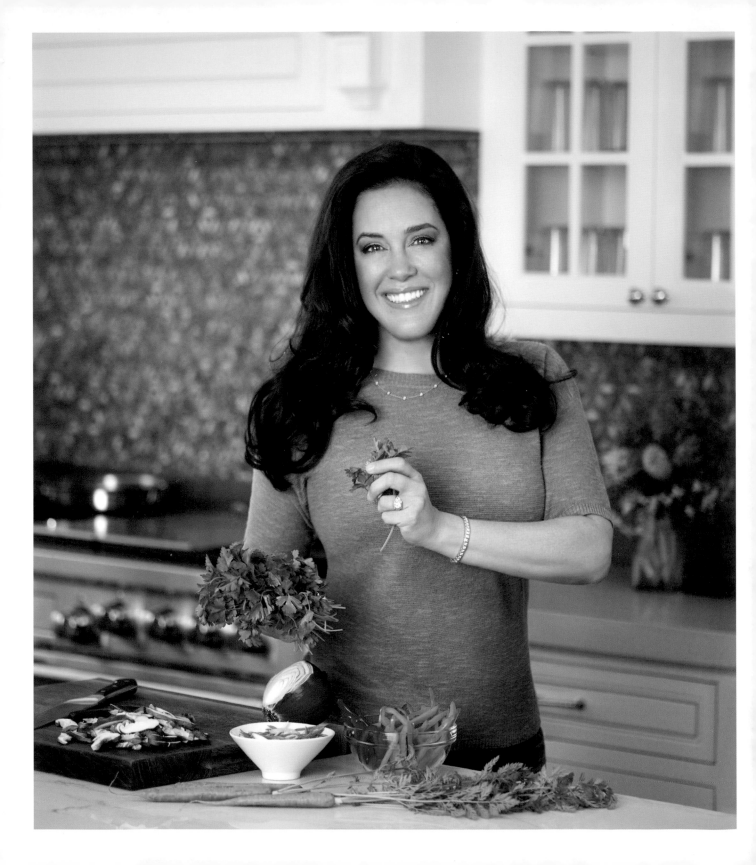

COOKING FOR A
FAST METABOLISM
Eat More Food and Lose More Weight

HAYLIE POMROY

WITH EVE ADAMSON

HOUGHTON MIFFLIN HARCOURT
BOSTON / NEW YORK / 2020

This book presents, among other things, the research and ideas of its author. It is not intended to be a substitute for consultation with a professional healthcare practitioner. Consult with your healthcare practitioner before starting any diet regimen. The publisher and the author disclaim responsibility for any adverse effects resulting directly or indirectly from information contained in this book.

Library of Congress Cataloging-in-Publication Data is available.
ISBN 978-0-358-16028-1 (POB);
ISBN 978-0-358-16029-8 (ebook)

Photography by Michael Hulswit and Aline Ponce
Book design by Rita Sowins

Printed in China
TOP 10 9 8 7 6 5 4 3 2 1

I DEDICATE THIS BOOK TO MY CHILDREN AND TO ALL THOSE WHO HAVE ENTERED MY KITCHEN. MAY YOU LEAVE FULL, BOTH IN YOUR BELLY AND IN YOUR HEART. THE NEED AND DESIRE FOR FOOD IS UNIVERSAL, AND AS WE BREAK BREAD TOGETHER, MAY THIS FOOD NOURISH YOU SO YOU MAY ENRICH OTHERS!

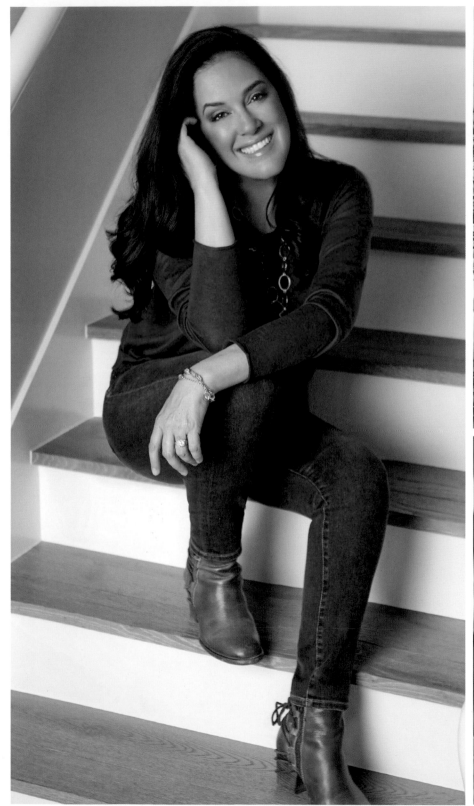
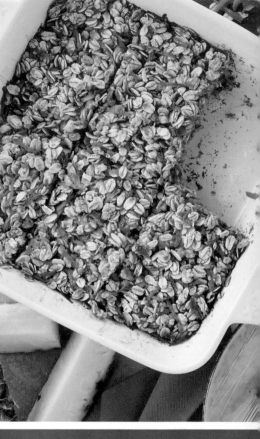
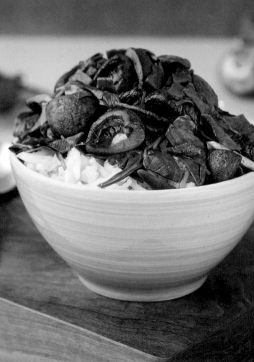

CONTENTS

INTRODUCTION

GROWING UP AS A KID WITH SEVERE FOOD ALLERGIES,
I began to distrust food in general at a young age. Whenever I ate the wrong thing, I would
get rashes on my lips and eyelids and eczema on my elbows and behind my knees. I spent
more time in soothing oatmeal baths than I did on the playground. It wasn't until college,
when I found myself in the hospital on 16 mg of prednisone, that a good friend introduced
me to a pioneer in integrative medicine, who she thought could help me. He reminded me
of the power of holistic medicine and natural foods, which I had grown up with but drifted
away from. He suggested I remove all sugar and processed foods from my diet and eat only
whole foods. My eczema disappeared! Food fixed something even powerful steroids hadn't
fixed, and that is when I recognized the direct correlation between my diet, my skin outbreaks,
and my overall health.

With the goal of minimizing my allergic reactions, my first experiments with cooking
were very basic, and the results were quite bland. I knew I had to be careful, but what I really
wanted was to enjoy my food. Whenever I ate out at restaurants, I loved the taste of the food,
but I hated what it did to my body. I wanted the food I made at home to be just as tasty, but
without the uncomfortable aftereffects, so I began experimenting with natural ingredients to
amplify the taste of the foods that were already making a noticeable, positive impact on my
health. My personal journey sparked my passion for making food that was both outrageously
healthy and incredibly pleasing. What saved my life became my life's work.

It's easy to forget what food really is and what it can do. Convenience and speed have
become such necessities in this fast-paced world, that spending evenings cooking compli-

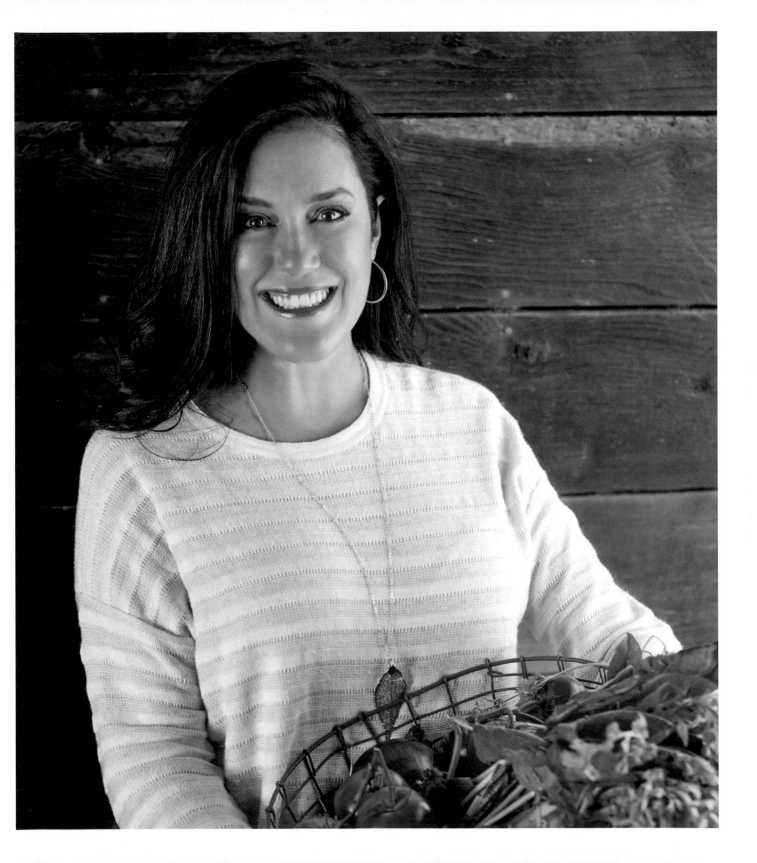

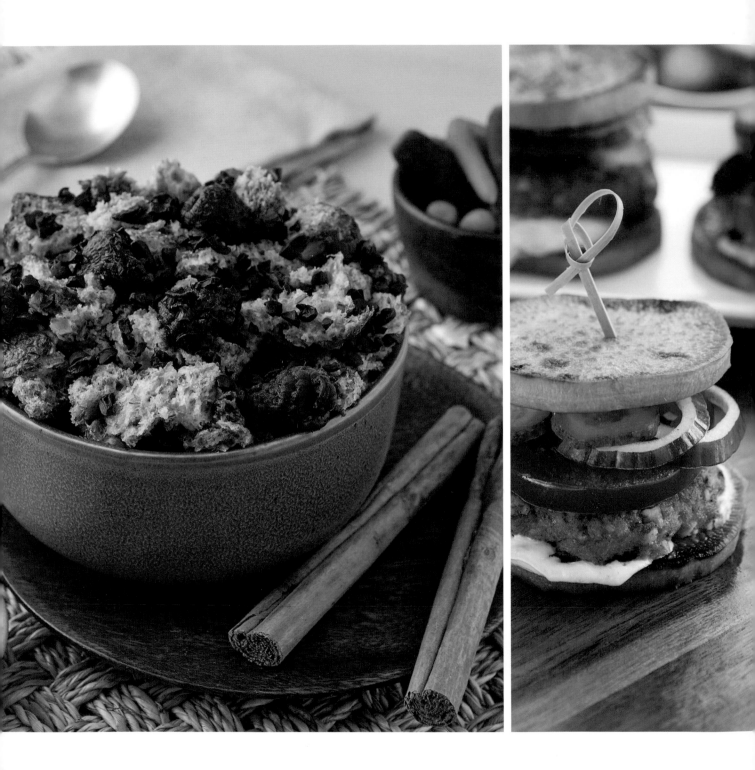

cated family dinners can seem foreign and unrealistic. But real, natural, whole-food cooking can be healthy and delicious—almost effortless. It can be a vibrant, exciting, comforting, energizing, calming, health-creating, even spiritual part of your life right here and now. For me, the kitchen is my pharmacy, my classroom, and the center of my family life. It's where we all do our homework, where we celebrate together, where we commune. I designed my kitchen for this purpose, and I spend most of my time at home in that space, cooking, experimenting, sharing, listening, laughing.

Don't get me wrong—I'm a businesswoman, a mother, an avid horseman, a scientist, a clinician. I'm busy just like you are. I don't want you to envision me slaving over a hot stove all day, my brow powdered with freshly ground flour. But that's not to say that I don't sometimes have multiple slow cookers and stockpots bubbling away in my kitchen, or that I don't sometimes feel inspired to cook multiple meals at once to be stored in stackable, labeled freezer containers. For me, prepping and consuming whole foods is a matter of life or death. I had to make peace with this reality first. Then, I completely fell in love with the whole process of finding the freshest, most natural foods, prepping them, cooking them, and freezing my own "fast food" so I always have something nourishing and delicious to eat. There are a lot of days when I just don't have time to do anything other than simply take something I made out of the freezer and reheat it.

The kitchen in my home is a place for delighting in food, not fearing it. Cooking has become a pleasure, not a chore. I wrote this cookbook to share that pleasure and the power and influence your kitchen can have over your health. Making a meal shouldn't be intimidating. It should be easy. Food shouldn't be a source of fear. It should be a source of love and a way to care for and nurture yourself and the people you care about. It can taste amazing while still being one of the most powerful tools you have in the defense of your own health. It can support your weight loss, as well as your efforts to improve your health and your mood.

But you won't find that kind of medicinal power in a package of processed food from a factory that you throw into the microwave and call a "meal." Real food comes from the earth, and in its healthiest form, it almost always requires some preparation. It doesn't have to take hours. Preparing your own food is a way to take care of yourself and keep your metabolism fired up or wake it up if it has slowed down.

What About Your Metabolism?

What is this "metabolism" you may have been hearing so much about, and what does it have to do with your weight loss and health goals? Basically, your metabolism is the process by which your body turns food into fuel or substance (like muscles, bones, skin, and blood). A fast metabolism stimulates the body toward restoration, not degeneration. For weight loss in particular, a fast metabolism means your body is efficiently converting food and fat into fuel. A fast metabolism can help to melt away fat, flatten your belly, trim your thighs, and un-jiggle your upper arms, as your body taps into the energy stores you have been holding onto (in the form of fat), maybe for years. On top of all that, a fast metabolism can help other processes in your body work more efficiently, easing your digestion, sharpening your thinking, boosting your mood, and giving you the energy you need to accomplish all the things you need to do every day.

And the way to make it all happen? With food! Food can hypernourish the metabolic pathways that regulate everything from inflammation to digestion to weight loss. Since every biochemical process going on inside you is micronutrient-dependent, a wide variety of whole foods will most likely touch all those bases, get all systems working efficiently, and keep your metabolism burning the way it's meant to burn.

Cooking for a Fast Metabolism

I have a dear friend, Kelly, who I asked to do the Fast Metabolism Diet (from my first book) along with me—she is my friend, after all. She had, in her words, "no cooking skills." Well, she lost more than 20 pounds, fell in love with food, and can now whip up a mean meal. She even meets with small groups, introducing them to the fast metabolism lifestyle, showing them how to make chili and pancakes and stack prepared meals in their freezers. One day she came to me and said her mom was struggling with her health. But she didn't want to put her mom on a diet program. She just wanted to figure out a way to make a positive impact in her mom's life through food. That's when the idea of this cookbook came to me.

I wanted to make something basic yet powerful that took almost no experience or introduction, not only for those who are already familiar with my plans and want more recipe options, but for those who aren't interested in doing any particular plan but want to transform their health simply by eating better food. I wanted to be able to have something that Kelly could give to her mom and, with confidence, say, "This is going to change your life." It's that simple—you don't have to be on a "plan" to change your health. All you have to do is get in the kitchen and learn how to use real, whole-food ingredients to transform your body, speed up your metabolism, and get all your systems working better. It really is that easy. The recipes in this book are designed to make an impact in your life any day and every day, at any meal and every meal, without complex cooking skills or kitchen intimidation.

Every single recipe in this book contains only foods from the Master Metabolism Food List—a list of the foods that fire up your metabolism rather than slow it down. Eat primarily from this list and you will be throwing kindling on your metabolism and flooding your body with the micronutrients it needs, even if you aren't following any particular eating plan.

In chapter one, you will find some powerful fast metabolism rules and information about how, when, and why to eat. In chapter two, for the first time in any of my books, I'm going to take you into my kitchen and show you some of the ideas I've implemented in my own home. I'm going to help you set up your kitchen, stock your pantry, and navigate the food list. You can use this list to maximize your experience with the recipes with nearly endless options for swapping out ingredients and tailoring recipes to your tastes and needs. You'll get guidance on substituting foods you don't like or can't have with those that work better for you, and information on portion sizes and servings. I'm going to help you plan your week and cook ahead for a month. And for anyone who is doing any of the plans from my other books, I have provided hints, tips, and cues for how to adapt these recipes to work along with whatever you are already doing for your metabolism. Whether you are on Phase 2 of the Fast Metabolism Diet, Part 1 of Metabolism Revolution, deep into the H-Burn, cleansing in preparation for the red carpet (or your next beach vacation) by doing my 5-Day red-carpet-ready cleanse, or are entirely new to my programs, you will find what you need in these pages. The Master Metabolism Food List will be a trusted reference to stoke your inner fire and flood your body with the micronutrients it needs to help you feel (and look) your best.

I also wanted to create a cookbook you could give to *your* friends, family, doctors, kids' teachers, or work colleagues that would offer an easy introduction to the Fast Metabolism lifestyle, in hopes that maybe they will prepare you something healthy the next time they invite you over (wink wink, hint hint)! I absolutely love it when someone says, "Come over for dinner. I made your Fast Metabolism Chili!" I get excited and my immune system lets out a huge sigh of relief. And I feel good knowing that the people in my life are feeding themselves well and nurturing their own health, too.

This is a cookbook you can use for the rest of your life in every aspect of your life. Although it isn't a weight loss cookbook, you can certainly use it for weight loss (and if you follow its principles, you are likely to lose weight without trying, if that's what you need). This isn't a holiday cookbook, but you can certainly use it for holidays—many of these recipes are worthy of the most splendid celebrations. This isn't a cookbook for any single one of my plans, but you can certainly use it in conjunction with my plans by following the guidance at the end of chapter two. This isn't a cookbook geared for special appliances or just one type of meal or food category or for any other narrow purpose—this is a lifelong cookbook that you can use in any situation, for any reason, or for no reason at all other than to fall in love with food again.

Breaking bread is a ceremonial thing people can do together. Some of my best memories are of cooking in the kitchen with my grandmother, who taught me how to poach an egg, and with my mother, who taught me how to flour a cube steak for the best chicken fried steak I've ever tasted. The photos in this cookbook are testimony to generations of family meals and kitchen communion. If you look on page 111, you'll see my grandmother's salt and pepper shakers, and on page 214 you can get a peek at the linens my mom inherited after my grandmother Gigi passed away and which I borrowed from her linen closet. That's Gigi's cast-iron skillet on page 214 and the muffin tins on page 259 came out of the trailer my grandparents hauled to the beach every year—I've diligently packed and unpacked them in various moves over the years. The dish holding the egg muffins on page 127 was a gift from one of my clients, and the chairs around my kitchen island were the heirlooms of another family who wanted to make sure their mother's special chairs found a warm and welcoming home.

In other words, the photos in this book show that my kitchen was created generationally. Every tool for food prep, every vessel for food delivery has its own story. The recipes and images in this book are a warm invitation into my kitchen and all of its history, which has shaped and informed my cooking over the years. Now that I'm a mother, I am passing these traditions and kitchen secrets along to my own children . . . and, through this book, to you.

My hope is that this book will help you discover the power of breaking bread together and creating a healthy life through healthy food with me, my community, and your own family and friends. I want to help you fill your kitchen with meaning as well as functionality. It doesn't matter whether your kitchen is big or small. It doesn't matter if your appliances are antique or ultra-modern. Your style of décor doesn't matter, and neither does the price of any of your tools. What matters is the intention behind and quality of the meals you prepare in that space—meals that can enrich both your health and your life and the health and lives of all the people you love.

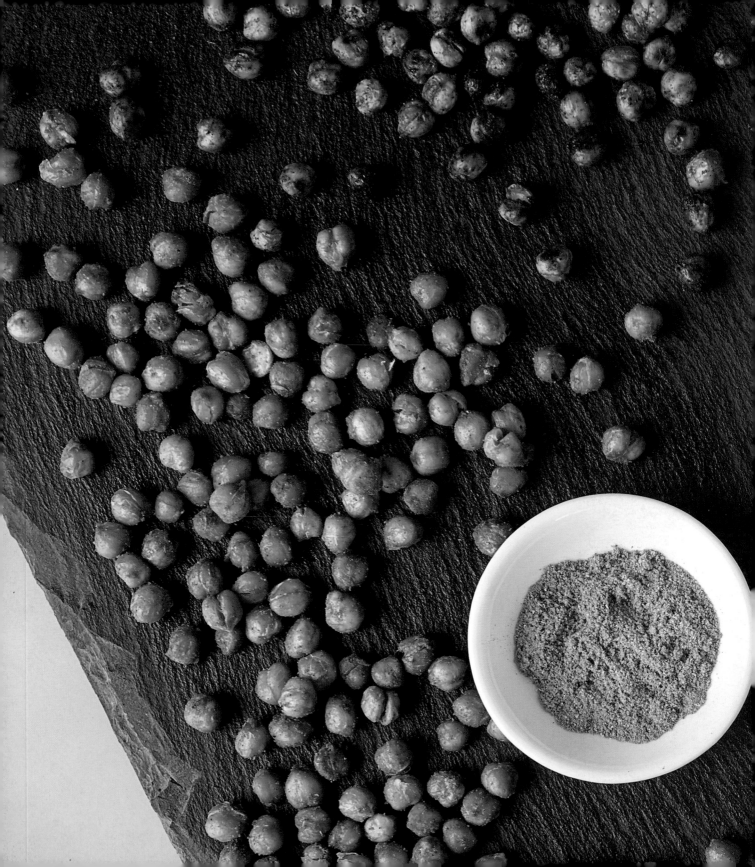

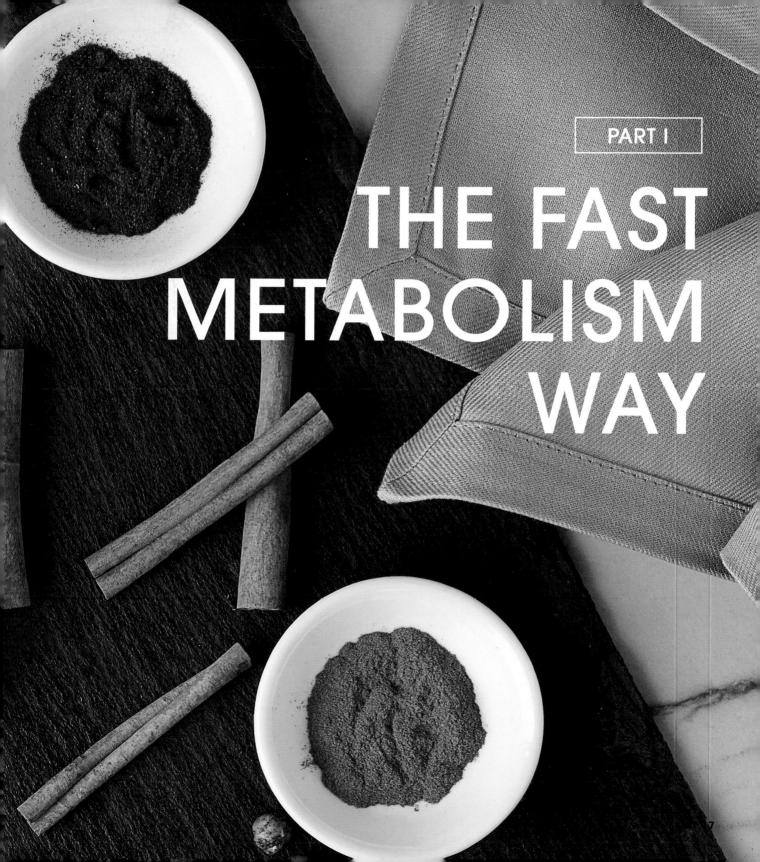

PART I

THE FAST METABOLISM WAY

IT TAKES DELICIOUS FOOD TO BUILD A FAST METABOLISM

Your body is a direct result of its environment, and that environment is largely shaped by food. What you eat and what you have eaten, how you live and how you have lived, what you do and what you have done, how you think and how you have thought, what you experience and what you have experienced, have all come together to create your body in its present state.

Have you spent years eating junk food? Chronically dieting? Depriving yourself, then binging when you can't take it anymore? Every one of these behaviors creates an environment to which your body has had to adapt via the resourceful and flexible nature of your metabolism. Not eating enough? Your metabolism slows down and saves all incoming energy for long-term survival. Experiencing chronic stress? Crisis hormones direct your body to store fat and burn muscle. Incoming junk food? Your body knows to seal it up in fat cells to protect you from those harmful pesticides and chemical preservatives. But if you manage your stress and eat real whole food most of the time, that body fat becomes a valuable fuel source, and your metabolism finally has the space and safety to rev up and use it. Burn, baby, burn!

Just as you are a product of your past, the body you will have tomorrow, next week, next month, next year, or ten, twenty, or fifty years from now is built from what you do from this day forward. What kind of body do you want to build? What kind of metabolism do you want to foster? What do you want to do with your fat stores? Keep them on your belly, butt, thighs, and arms? Or do you want to burn them off to reveal a stronger, more energetic you? In other words: What kind of future do you want for yourself?

You've got a lot of power on your plate and plenty of opportunity to manifest the body and life of your dreams. And while you can't control every aspect of your environment, there is one thing you have more control over than anything else: what you eat.

I have published many books containing many different plans and programs for addressing a variety of different issues, from breaking weight loss plateaus to remedying chronic health issues, achieving rapid weight loss, cleansing, and more. That's because from day to day, the demands and expectations you put on your body vary drastically. You may be going through extreme stress (which can be physical, mental, or emotional);

looking to lose weight; or wanting to improve your mood, naturally metabolize cholesterol, or stabilize your blood sugar. In each of these scenarios, your needs will be different. But they do have one thing in common: You can achieve all those goals and more through food.

My plans aren't diets—at least, not in the sense of the word you may be familiar with. Each of my programs acts as a playbook to keep you winning on the field of life. You are the team captain, and by bringing a nutritionist on board—me—you will acquire the skill set to slice and dice, sauté and bake, broil and stir-fry your way to becoming a master of your kitchen and your health.

There is no more pressing time than now to master the fine art of cooking and eating real food in a strategic way. Chronic disease has reached epidemic proportions—the growth of the health care sector is proof of this increasingly urgent problem. Did you know that the largest real estate growth in this country is health care related—hospitals, eldercare, physical rehabilitation centers, mental health centers? People are seeking help when their health declines, but many find themselves navigating their wellness care alone, until their imbalances and issues have progressed to a dire state.

But with a commitment to a healthy lifestyle now, you can avoid ever getting to that place. With a nutritionist in your life, you can learn what works for you. You'll learn how to spin plans, modify recipes, and accumulate valuable knowledge about your health, your body, and how to make it all work for you. Even though you don't know it all yet (even *I* don't know it all yet!), you'll learn what questions to ask. You'll become aware of your knowledge gaps, and you'll discover how much there is to know about how to curate your lifestyle to promote your own wellness.

Just by buying this book, you become part of the community of people who have worked through my plans to address specific issues and who have embraced fast metabolism living. We share with each other, we swap recipes and cooking techniques, we support each other—we are a tribe, and we would love to engage with you and welcome you into our midst. We have a private membership group where people can ask us questions, help each other out, and share their secrets, tips, and triumphs. Every time I hear another success story, I'm amazed at how far people in our community have come. People who used to hate going to the grocery store or were afraid of cooking have evolved into experienced cooks who know how to use food to maximize their own health and lives. They are making, eating, and adoring the food that is specific to their body's metabolic needs.

Tara is a good example. Tara joined our community not knowing how to do more than heat up a premade microwave meal. Now she speaks the fast metabolism language, pulling aspects from each of my plans to harness the micronutrient power of food. Not only has she lost more than forty pounds, she now has the energy and sass to be the master of her own metabolism. This can be you, and we welcome you with open arms. This cookbook is for you so you will never have to wonder what to eat. With the Master Metabolism Food List, you won't have to ask, "Will this food fuel my metabolism?" You'll already know the answer is "Yes!" You can shape any recipe to meet your current needs and be compliant with any plan you choose to follow. This book can be a catalyst for changing your life. You have a nutritionist now—you no longer have to navigate this field alone.

D.I.E.T. = Did I Eat Today?

I believe strongly that the only way to speed up your metabolism is not to diet (in the sense of deprivation), but to eat. Yes, you actually need to *eat more* (of the right foods) to lose more weight. It seems counterintuitive, but I know from decades of experience that this is how it works.

The reason you need to eat is to support your metabolism. When you have a fast metabolism, you not only burn fat more efficiently, but you do everything more efficiently, like build muscle, grow shiny hair and strong nails, develop healthy skin and robust collagen, manufacture energy, and fuel weight loss. But the metabolism needs fuel to run, and *food is the fuel.* This is why I believe it is so important to D.I.E.T. rather than "diet."

In my world and in our community, D.I.E.T. means "Did I Eat Today?" I ask myself this question every day, and I suggest you do, too. Did you eat the foods today that will get you healthy and keep you healthy? Did you eat the foods that give you energy and drive? Did you eat the foods that make you look and feel amazing, like you can take on the world? Even if you don't know which foods those are right now, you'll find the answers here.

Eating is the path to better health, even to a better life. What do you see when you think about the life you desire? I tell my clients—and you're one of them now, too—to dream big. I have overcome major health challenges simply by eating—and I attribute the power on my plate to much of the health and life success I've had. It all starts with that question: "Did I Eat Today?" Ask yourself, "Did I eat today to achieve the life I desire?" When you ask yourself that question, I want you to be able to answer, "Oh yes, I did! And it was a delicious experience."

The D.I.E.T. Dozen

Before we get into the specific foods, I want to share some basic practices for eating that I give to all my clients. For maximum metabolic benefit, here are your D.I.E.T. guidelines:

1. Always eat within 30 minutes of waking. If you don't have time for breakfast, at least have a snack. Science tells us that morning fasting, i.e., not eating within 30 minutes of waking, is stressful on the body. Most of us have busy mornings. How can our bodies

drive us through everything we need to do without any fuel? Not eating when your body needs fuel causes the adrenal glands to secrete the stress hormone cortisol and other famine hormones that promote weight gain—specifically by accumulating and storing fat in the belly and thigh areas. To mobilize that fat and burn it, fuel your metabolism first thing every morning!

2. Always eat five times every day—three meals and two snacks. No skipping! Keep the fires stoked. The micronutrients from food make the metabolism functional.

3. Eat every three to four hours, except when you are sleeping. This is very important for creating a consistent and stable blood glucose level, inhibiting surges of insulin that can slow the body's natural metabolic rate.

4. Eat organic, seasonal, and/or local food whenever possible. The fresher and more naturally grown your food is, the more nutrient-dense it is. Those nutrients are responsible for keeping the biochemistry of your metabolism optimized and stable without the added burden of pesticides, herbicides, and preservatives.

5. Variety is the spice of life. Don't eat any recipe more than three times per week. Not only does mixing up your meals help to heal food allergies and sensitivities from overexposure to certain foods, but it also makes a significant difference in metabolic efficiency, which is driven by micronutrients. Our bodies are biodiverse organisms undergoing a constant barrage of stressors and burdens, and diversifying your food over the course of a week helps to level the playing field. Some of the primary things food diversity will do for you are:

   - Provide you with more phytonutrients, including vitamins, minerals, hormone precursors, antioxidants, pro- and prebiotics, amino acids, and other health-promoting plant substances.
   - Expose you to more enzymes, which help you to digest the diverse foods you choose. For example, a food higher in fat will stimulate the gallbladder and liver to produce bile salts for fat digestion. A food heavier in complex carbohydrates will stimulate the pancreas to produce healthy levels of insulin to assimilate those sugars.

A food heavier in protein will stimulate the stomach to produce more hydrochloric acid and the pancreas to produce more protease, for more efficient protein digestion.

- Improve your hormone production, absorption, and utilization. Hormones aren't just estrogen, progesterone, and testosterone. They also include many secretory hormones that regulate fat metabolism, the development of lean muscle, and the stabilization of blood sugar (insulin is a hormone); help us feel full and satisfied after eating; reduce and regulate cravings; and more. Hormones are the mechanism by which the body adapts to its environment and achieves homeostasis (balance).
- Support your microflora, or the good bacteria that make up your internal ecosystem (what some people call the gut biome or microbiome). Your gut bacteria help to assimilate nutrients such as B vitamins, prevent yeast overgrowth, inhibit bad bacterial colonization, stabilize blood pH, and aid in the production and absorption of mood-elevating neurotransmitters like serotonin.

Now *that* is a lot of power on your plate!

6. Drink half your body weight in ounces of spring water every day. Dilution is the solution for pollution! Science shows us that fat-soluble toxins not only slow our rate of burn but can create a host of diseases, ranging from neurological to autoimmune.

7. If it's fake, huge mistake! Avoid all highly processed, chemically laden "food." Many of us in the nutrition industry are attempting to get approximately 50 percent of what is on the labels of processed food to not be allowed to be sold as food because, by definition, these substances are not food. These are chemicals used to add pigment to paint, strengthen bulletproof vests, and kill weeds and bugs. They have no business going in your mouth.

8. Exercise, but eat something first. Have at least a snack before a workout. You need to give your body something to run on. I always say, "Don't fast before going fast." Although you may have heard that you should exercise before eating anything, I strongly disagree with this advice. Our bodies are designed to adapt to our environments and circumstances, and because exercise is a stressor to the body (albeit a positive one, in most cases), the body has to adapt to it and adjust to its effects, including post-exercise

repair. When you stress the body and the body doesn't sense that there is an abundance of nutrients for repair on board, it will extract glucose from the muscles and the liver, minerals from the bones, and bile salts from the digestive tract in order to prepare for and begin the repair process. This begins the second the body senses an increase in the contraction and relaxation of the muscles—in other words, the second you start exercising. If you've eaten something first, the body won't have to cannibalize your various resources and can focus instead on giving you the energy you need and laying down stronger lean muscle in response to your physical activity.

9. Pleasure stimulates the metabolism. Savor and enjoy your meals without guilt! A cascade of hormones is released when you eat. A healthy cascade happens when it's a positive experience, and an unhealthy cascade happens when there is stress surrounding a meal.

10. Cooking is fun. It doesn't have to be hard or messy. It can be easy and convenient. You'll see! (Did I mention pleasure stimulates the metabolism? Well, that fun can begin in the kitchen.)

11. Plan your meals. Planning is paramount. In every aspect of life, when you define your destination, it's much easier to chart your path forward. In this book, I'll help you create your own unique and strategic meal maps based on what you want to achieve with your metabolism.

12. Finally, never forget to ask yourself the fundamental question: Did I eat today? Did I eat to achieve the health, the energy, the sleep, the joy, and the enjoyment that I deserve?

If you can integrate the D.I.E.T. Dozen into your daily life, you are well on your way to a scorching metabolism!

What the Heck *Is* the Metabolism, Anyway?

If you're new to the fast metabolism way of life, you may be wondering what it is, exactly. Metabolism is a process, not a thing. Specifically, the metabolic process consists of chemical and biochemical reactions that occur in the cells of all living organisms to sustain life. It's the change or transformation of food into either heat and fuel or substance (muscle, fat, blood, bone). At any given moment, your metabolism is either burning, storing, or building.

Your metabolism affects every single aspect of your life. It affects how strong your bones are, how shiny your hair is, how firm and tight your skin looks, how strong your nails are, how solid your tendons and ligaments are, how good your mood is, how well your immune system functions, how much stress hormone is circulating through your system at any given moment, how well you process cholesterol and sugar, how sharp your memory stays, even how much of a sex drive you have. Metabolism is the process by which your body takes food in and transforms it for its own use—for energy, rebuilding, repairing, restoring, growing, moving, and all-around living.

But *your* metabolism doesn't work exactly like anyone else's. It constantly adjusts for your unique body living in your unique environment. Every time your environment changes, your metabolism shifts to accommodate that change. It is constantly dynamic and never static, because your biochemistry is constantly in flux, too. But it can't do what it needs to do without input: food, rest, and movement. Your metabolism is capable of being incredibly agile and responsive, but only if you provide it with the raw materials it needs. Your metabolism is largely shaped by what you give it, and it has to take what it gets and make the best of it.

E + M = H

This simple equation breaks down why it is so important to give your metabolism what it needs.

E: EATING, EXERCISE, ENVIRONMENT

+

M: METABOLISM, METABOLIC PATHWAYS, "ME" (THAT MEANS YOU!)

=

H: HEALTH, HOMEOSTASIS, HARMONY

What this means is that what you eat, how you much exercise, and your environment (both internal and external) added to the action of your metabolism, the effectiveness of your metabolic pathways, and everything within you ("me") that generates life determine how healthy you are, how well your body is able to maintain homeostasis, and your biological state of harmony.

The most important thing to understand about this equation is the E, because *you can control the E*, which influences the M, which determines the H. Your choices about what and how you eat, how much and whether you exercise, and what kind of environment you are in are the start. Your next meal is part of this equation. Everything you do is plugged into this formula, which is why your actions today dictate the quality of your life tomorrow.

Metabolism Myths and Facts

Metabolism is complex, and that might be why there are so many misconceptions about it, like "You lose weight by not eating." (Actually, you lose weight *by eating.*) Or, "You have diabetes because you eat sugar." (Actually, you have diabetes because you can't metabolize sugar.) Or, "You have high cholesterol because you eat cholesterol." (Actually, you have high cholesterol because you aren't metabolizing cholesterol efficiently.) Or, "You're in a bad mood because you're 'hangry.'" (That's hunger that makes you angry!) (Actually, you're in a bad mood because you don't have the nutrient reserves to keep your adaptogenic hormones balanced during times of extreme stress.)

I want to dispel these misconceptions because, for so many of us, they have taught us to turn away from food instead of toward it. Let's set the record straight and dispel these four metabolic myths.

Myth #1: The Way to Lose Weight Is to Eat Less

This is probably the most pervasive myth out there and one of the most dangerous. There is no more efficient way to slow down your metabolism and increase your risk of excessive weight gain than dieting. I have had many, many clients over the years come to me confused and frustrated because they severely limit their calories but their weight remains higher than is comfortable for them. Many of them also exercise, sometimes daily. But they can't lose the unwanted weight!

Metabolism is nutrient dependent, which means fuel from food is what determines the rate of burn. This is why you *must* eat strategically to stimulate the metabolism and to have a fast metabolism. Starvation will slow your rate of burn over time. When you don't eat but work hard all day, even exercise, your body has to find energy somewhere, and the body is resourceful. That's when it begins to feast on your own muscle tissue (this is called *catabolism*—metabolism's evil twin). Not only will you be unable to build muscle from exercise, but you will lose muscle, and exercise will stress your body rather than benefit it. When those stress hormones start flowing, your body stores fat aggressively— even from celery!

People are often surprised that they can gain weight from foods like celery and lettuce, but I've seen it happen many times. Our bodies are designed for survival. During stressful times, the body conserves potential energy (i.e., fat) and uses it sparingly. When there seems to be no end in sight to chronic stress, the body conserves its resources. Even though we may feel that fat is unsightly or uncomfortable, the body sees it as a lifesaving resource. The more your body feels in crisis, the more it's going to hoard its resources, and that means that *any* incoming food can be stored as fat. The less you eat, the worse it gets. The only way to turn this situation around is to eat *more*, so your metabolism has fuel again and can restart, burning what you eat instead of burning your muscle tissue and aggressively storing incoming food as fat. I will always encourage you to stoke the fire, and the kindling is food.

Myth #2: If It's Delicious, It's Naughty

Here's a wonderful fact about the metabolism: Pleasure is slimming. When you enjoy your food, you reduce your stress hormones and give your body permission to burn fat. Eating bland "diet food" you don't like is stressful and unsatisfying. Stress is fattening. Food is meant to be beautiful, delicious, natural. I want you to revel in it, to fall in love with it all over again. When you make peace with food, your metabolism thrives.

Myth #3: Calories Are Worth Counting

This is another big myth: that calories are something that can actually be measured or that they should be counted at all. The truth is, calories are a lie. They have very little to do with how your body responds to food. You'll be able to convince me that Bigfoot exists or the moon landing was a hoax before you'll convince me that calories are relevant. Calories are a marketing tool and nothing more.

Do you know how they determine calories? They put a food in a sealed container and put the container in water. Then they burn the food to ash. A calorie is the amount of energy required to raise the temperature of 1 kilogram of water by 1°C when the food is burned. Talk about theoretical. Do you really think if a 20-pound toddler eats a granola bar and metabolizes it for energy, that toddler will get the same amount of energy from it as a 250-pound body builder would? Of course not. That's like saying it takes the same amount of energy for a toddler to lift a 10-pound weight off the ground as it takes for that body builder to lift that 10-pound weight off the ground. The truth is, that body builder could lift the weight *and* the toddler and still expend a fraction of the energy the toddler had to expend trying to pick up that big dumbbell.

So what about that whole "2,000 calories a day" rule we've all been taught to live by? The fact is, it's really kind of embarrassing for anyone who actually understands anything about biochemistry, chemistry, or the diversity of humankind—the person to the right or left of you is nothing like you!—that this false belief has become so prevalent. Calories are a chemistry experiment, and while I'll admit that the body itself is one big science experiment, it actually works very differently than the calorie experiment would have us believe. I will never tell you that eating should resemble anything like adding or deducting from a bank account.

So forget counting calories. They have nothing to do with you or your metabolism, and they're certainly not the answer for getting your body and your health where you want them to be.

Myth #4: You're Not Healthy Because You Eat Too Many Desserts

Guilt is as bad for your metabolism as stress is. Enjoy what you're eating, whatever it may be. If you adopt this new concept, you will have a much better chance of secreting hormones that stabilize blood sugar and build bone, muscle, ligaments, and health. By extracting every and any valuable micronutrient from that food (as long as it is actually food), you will help your metabolism. We do not gain weight because we eat dessert. If we gain weight from a dessert, it's because we can't metabolize the dessert we are eating. We all know that person who can eat anything and not gain an ounce of weight. They have a higher rate of burn, plain and simple. The goal—not just because it affects weight but because it affects aspects of health in the body—is to have the most efficient metabolism possible. If yours isn't (yet) as efficient as it could be, don't blame dessert. Instead, listen carefully to your body and be in awe of its ability to repair your metabolism. In my book, desserts can be created with the implicit intention of promoting health. All that being said, refined sugar and refined carbohydrates, as well as food additives like food coloring and chemicals, can have a negative health impact that reaches far beyond mere weight gain. So while a packaged, processed dessert made with packaged, processed ingredients is no good for your metabolism, a dessert made with whole foods in your own kitchen is sheer pleasure. Once your metabolism is repaired and efficient at burning food for fuel, you can indulge in *that* kind of dessert regularly, with pleasure and without guilt.

So What Is Food, Anyway?

As long as we're on the subject of dessert, what is food, exactly? And by that, I mean what is *real* food? Food is something that was once alive and came from the land, sky, or sea. An apple is food. Blueberries are food. So are chickens and sweet potatoes, salmon and mangoes, avocados and almonds, oats and oranges, carrots and cucumbers, and crisp, leafy greens.

But here's what's *not* food:

- Artificial colors like Blue #2, Yellow #6, and Red #40.
- Artificial preservatives like sodium benzoate, sodium sulfite, sodium nitrate, and butylated hydroxytoluene (try saying that three times fast!).
- Artificial sweeteners like aspartame and saccharin.
- Flavor enhancers like monosodium glutamate.
- Food additives like potassium bromate, sulfur dioxide, and propylene glycol.

- Pesticides like glyphosate and chlorpyrifos.
- Antibiotics like penicillin and enrofloxacin.
- Anything that was once alive but has been so heavily processed, mutated, or contaminated with these non-food substances that it is no longer recognizable as food—like high-fructose corn syrup, white sugar, trans fat, or even things as seemingly benign as a box of bright-colored sugary kid's cereal, a frozen package of deep-fried "chicken fingers" (what?), a microwavable diet dinner, or a "fun-size" bag of colorful candy (which is anything but fun for your metabolism). These highly processed "foods" are mere shadows of their former selves, ruined by modern industry. I would even call them abominations.

Dangerous Dozen

Before I send you off to the market with a shopping list or into the kitchen with a great recipe, let's look at what foods not to buy, or cook with, or eat because of their metabolism-inhibiting effects. In all my books, all my programs, and all the meal maps I create for my clients, I intentionally leave these twelve foods off my lists. Because you are my client now, I want you to know why. I call them the Dangerous Dozen. Here's what to keep out of your kitchen for maximized metabolism stoking:

1. **WHEAT:** You may have visions of golden stalks of wheat waving in the sun on a family farm in the great American Midwest, but I've got news for you: Wheat is a billion-dollar agricultural business, and over the centuries, in order to increase profit and yield, crop scientists have hybridized wheat so it can withstand extreme weather, pests, and pesticide application and still produce chunky grains full of starch. This has made wheat not just indestructible but mostly indigestible. If a heat wave or a plague of locusts can't take down a wheat plant, how is your stomach acid supposed to handle the task? It can't. That's why wheat can cause bloating, gas, water retention, fatigue, and inflammation in the body, even when you don't necessarily feel it (your body is used to steeling itself against wheat, and you may not realize how bad it makes you feel until you stop eating it). I have nothing against good natural whole-grain foods like brown and wild rice, barley, and quinoa. Even sprouted wheat is okay by me. But regular industrially produced wheat—including wheat flour and everything

made with it (most packaged bread, tortillas, bagels, English muffins, cookies, cake, etc.)—is a metabolism killer.

2. **CORN:** Corn is one of the worst things you can eat if you want to speed up your metabolism. As with wheat, corn has been drastically hybridized and modified, so it is difficult to digest. It's also been bred to be bigger, starchier, and sweeter, but even heirloom varieties and feed corn contain a carbohydrate structure that specifically encourages fat accumulation. When repairing the metabolism, I do not recommend any corn products. In my clinical setting, I do use corn when I have clients who aren't able to gain weight; I use corn as a catalyst for weight gain because corn's most impressive quality is to fatten. When farmers want to make sure their beef is "marbled" (meaning the muscles are full of white fat tissue), corn is their secret weapon. They feed the cows large amounts of corn right before slaughter. It's also what horses are often fed before a show if they've dropped too much weight. In other words, if you want to put on fat *fast*, corn is your answer.

3. **DAIRY:** You love cheese. I know. You could *never give up cheese.* I've heard it all before hundreds of times. But the sugar-fat-protein ratio in cheese and all other dairy products stimulates sex hormones in a way that tends to stall the metabolism. Organic whole milk can be a useful tool for fertility, but if you aren't trying to get pregnant, you're better off avoiding it. And forget the low-fat and fat-free versions. These are so high in sugar that they aggressively slow fat metabolism.

4. **SOY:** If you don't eat animal protein, organic, non–genetically modified (GMO), mini-mally processed soy like fresh tofu, edamame, and tempeh can be good sources of protein. However, most soy is heavily processed (if you see "soy protein isolate" on an ingredients list, step away), and soy is one of the most genetically modified crops, making it difficult for the body to break down. Also, even organic soy contains phytoes-trogens, which are plant compounds that have an estrogen-like effect in the body. I know of no better way to increase belly fat than by eating soy. It's also used as a filler in livestock feed (much in the same way that the food industry adds soy protein to hamburgers and many other processed foods—it's cheap protein). If you want to gain weight fast and slow your metabolism, dig into a big fat soy burger or a "veggie hot

dog." But don't worry, vegetarians—I've got plenty of high-protein meat-free foods for you. (Note: Exceptions to the no-soy rule include tamari and liquid aminos. Because they are extracted from fermented soy products, their estrogenic factors have been mostly neutralized.)

5. **REFINED SWEETENERS:** You throw a spoonful of sugar into your coffee or on top of your oatmeal in the morning—so what? A lot happens, actually, even from very little. Refined sugar is a highly concentrated source of quick energy, but even a tiny bit more than your body can use becomes very difficult for your body to process. To prevent your blood sugar from getting too high, your body directs that excess sugar right into your fat cells. When you eat too many cookies, you're basically swelling your fat cells. Just two teaspoons of refined sugar can inhibit your weight loss for three to four days. Think about that the next time you contemplate that jumbo root beer at the movie theater or that slab of birthday cake. You might decide it's worth it, but if you're working on losing weight, the price you pay will be a stalled number on the scale.

Also, refined sugars are often combined with glycoprotein from pig's blood or bone char, which makes refined sugar even more fattening and addictive. Glycoprotein inhibits insulin's effectiveness at sending sugar into the cells to be burned. The result is that sugar in the blood remains elevated. This is a dangerous situation. Sustained elevated blood sugar levels can cause neurologic and immune damage, so to protect you, your body stimulates the activation and creation of more adipocytes (fat cells) to absorb the increased glucose in the blood. The body creates fat cells in order to protect you.

So why do they add glycoprotein to sugar? One of the reasons is that glycoprotein triggers a cascade of brain reactions that make you crave more sugar. As I've explained, sugar should go into the cells to be burned, and when this works, the brain gets the message that the body doesn't need any more sugar. But if the sugar isn't shuttled into the fat cells, the brain becomes ravenous for sugar, thinking it isn't getting enough because the cells aren't getting enough. So, adding glycoproteins is a tricky way to stimulate addiction to particular foods. (Thank you for joining me in this science-geek moment!) And, on top of all of that, both glycoprotein and bone char turn refined white sugar into a product that is definitely *not* vegetarian (in case that is a concern for you).

6. **CAFFEINE:** If you love your coffee, here's some good news: Coffee itself doesn't cause weight gain. However, it's not part of the program for healing the metabolism because caffeine is hard on your adrenal glands, which produce stress hormones like aldosterone and cortisol. To your adrenal glands, a cup of coffee feels like *stress*, which triggers the release of aldosterone and cortisol, which then interfere with efficient metabolic function. Think of it this way: Running a marathon doesn't break your bones, but if you have a broken bone, you shouldn't run a marathon. Drinking coffee is like running a marathon. If your metabolism is slow, that's like having a broken bone. So abstain from caffeine while healing your metabolism. Once your metabolism is running fast and efficiently, you may be able to handle the occasional cup of coffee (but keep it organic—conventional coffee is one of the most heavily sprayed crops and is full of chemical residue). If you are in the coffee habit, you may feel grumpy or headachy for a few days, but as soon as you step out of that caffeine fog, you'll experience renewed energy and an amazing feeling of well-being, better than any caffeine buzz. That good feeling is your body operating the way it's meant to—providing you with natural energy rather than stress-fueled energy. Also avoid decaf, which still has some caffeine. (And if this is a deal breaker for you, my advice is to choose only organic low-acid coffee and to never, ever drink it unless you eat something first.) The same goes for black, green, and white teas. Some kinds of tea don't have as much caffeine as coffee, but any caffeine, especially without food first, is a metabolism killer.

---

7. **ALCOHOL:** You may like to enjoy a glass of wine to destress after a long workday, or maybe you like a beer with dinner or a cocktail when you go out on the town. I get that! But before you swill yet another drink, just know that alcohol, like any other toxin, must be processed through your liver. When you drink alcohol, your liver's first priority will become to protect you. When you're trying to lose weight and regain your health, your liver function is a key player. The liver is responsible for converting thyroid hormones into an active state. It also converts the fat molecule cholesterol into sex hormones and makes them bioavailable. On top of all that, it's the most important organism in the body's natural detoxification process. Because the liver is so significant in so many areas directly related to weight loss, the more stress you can take off the liver, the more efficiently it can help your body burn fat. And we all know that too much alcohol stresses the liver. Even one drink will distract your body's detoxification

system and fat metabolism from weight loss. Moreover, alcohol has loads of sugar, even if it says 0 carbs and 0 sugar when you look up something like vodka or gin on an online calorie counter. Alcohol is complex in this way—during metabolism, alcohol is converted to sugar through the liver, so the by-product of alcohol metabolism is sugar. This further stalls your metabolism as your body gets busy trying to keep your blood sugar in a safe range (rather than burning fat). For all these reasons, when you're working on weight loss, it's best to avoid alcohol or at least be prepared not to lose any weight until the alcohol has been processed out of your system.

8. **CHEMICALLY CURED MEAT:** Most deli meat, bacon, sausage, ham, bologna, hot dogs, and other cured meats are treated with nitrates and nitrites. These preservatives are added to prevent the food from spoiling, but the way that this is accomplished is by preventing the breakdown of the fat within these high-fat meats. Guess what happens in your body when you then consume these chemicals? They prevent the breakdown of fat in *your body*. If your priority is to break down and burn off your fat, nitrates and nitrites are not your friends. But you can still enjoy convenient deli meat. Just look for those labeled "nitrate-free" and "naturally cured." (And no sugar added!) Organic meats cannot contain nitrates or nitrites. Do keep in mind that deli meat without preservatives will not keep as long, however (no real food will keep all that long, which is an indicator that it is natural), so eat it within a couple of days or freeze it until you're ready to eat it.

9. **DRIED FRUIT/FRUIT JUICE:** Dried fruit can be as sweet as candy, and varieties without added sugar can be a good source of energy, especially if you're exercising hard. But most of the time, the sugar concentration in dried fruit is just too high. Fruit juice is also high in sugar, with none of the fiber from the whole fruit to slow down its absorption. Juice in particular will cause a surge in the delivery of sugar to your bloodstream. Once your metabolism is burning hot, you can enjoy a little dried fruit or a small glass of juice once in a while without bad effect (especially before a workout), but until then, it's best to avoid them.

10. **ARTIFICIAL SWEETENERS:** You already know that artificial sweeteners are not real food. They're chemicals made to trick your body into thinking it's getting sugar but that don't deliver any legitimate energy. Artificial sweeteners are literal poisons for

your body. They are officially classified as known obesegens, meaning they promote the hormones that contribute to obesity. They're also fat soluble, so when the body can't metabolize them, it stores them in fat pockets. The more you consume, the more fat you'll need to store them. Artificial sweeteners also stress the liver—remember, this organ is very important for detoxification and fat metabolism. Science has clearly demonstrated that artificial sweeteners disrupt the balance of your gut bacteria, promoting bacteria that is more conducive to weight gain and obesity. Finally, all artificial, synthetic sweeteners are known neurotoxins that disrupt enzyme production, destabilize blood sugar, and disrupt hormone-receptor sites. Considering how extensively some of these sweeteners have been researched, it's shocking that they are still available to consumers. All that toxicity with no payoff? I wouldn't get anywhere near them.

11. **FAT-FREE "DIET" FOODS:** I always say, "If it's fake, take a break," and that especially applies to packaged, processed "diet foods." Convenience is great, but there are much better ways to get a quick meal or snack. If it says "free," don't buy it. That little word "free" is a potent marketing tool. You should be aware that the majority of products that say they are "free" of something have some kind of artificial sweetener or addictive flavoring component added that will make your body crave these products. "Sugar-free" foods typically have artificial sweeteners to replicate that sweet taste experience, and "fat-free" foods typically have chemicals added to replicate the creamy texture of fat. But as soon as you take the natural fat or sugar out of a real food, you've turned it into something else your metabolism will have to try to decipher and, in many cases, that your liver will have to work to protect you from. That even goes for products that say "gluten-free." It's buyer beware. Turn the package around and read the label! A lot of products have jumped on the gluten-free marketing train, but many of those products contain obesegens and other metabolism killers that have been added to make these foods both palatable and addictive. There are plenty of fresh, real-food alternatives that are just as easy and taste so much better. Typically, the marketing behind nutrient-dense food features what they *do* contain, not what they don't contain.

12. **FASTING:** Fasting, especially what is popularly called "intermittent fasting," has become trendy lately. I consider this trend unsafe. Why subject your body to work, exercise, action, and thought without providing it with any fuel? Your muscles, your

organs, and especially your brain need fuel to function. This is why I ask you to eat your first meal or snack within 30 minutes of waking and then eat every three to four hours during the day. When your metabolism is slow, you are literally starving at a cellular level. The answer is not to starve more. And if you have blood sugar issues (such as metabolic syndrome, prediabetes, or diabetes), fasting is actually dangerous. If you experience a legitimate famine, your body does have ways to help get you through it, but that means shutting down many important systems for the sake of survival. I don't want you to survive. I want you to thrive, and that means I want you to eat food!

Whole-Food Broad Strokes: How Do You Pull It All Together?

There is healthy, and there is health strategy. They aren't exactly the same, but this book contains the information you need to accomplish both. Eating from the Master Metabolism Food List is the path to health, but following a strategic eating plan for a specific purpose is a health strategy. I have many plans for many purposes, and if you've been with me for a while, you know this. But if you're new to the fast metabolism lifestyle, you may be wondering what all these different plans are and maybe also wondering why there needs to be more than one plan. If one works, isn't that enough?

Some of my clients have been with me for twenty years, and it's not because every time they walk in the door, I give them the same plan. We look forward, we look backward, we talk about what they've been exposed to, what they're experiencing, what's coming next. Then we determine what they need in the snapshot that is their life at the current moment.

People gain weight or have trouble losing it for many reasons, and there are even more ways to customize meals and snacks to address those reasons. Some of my plans provide the means to lose a lot of weight over time, while others aim to help you lose weight *fast*. Some of my plans help break weight loss plateaus due to inflammation, digestive issues, or hormonal imbalances. Some help address particular health concerns.

But the one thing all my plans have in common is that they use specific foods in specific ways to strategically fire up your metabolism, reboot your weight loss, support your health goals, and grant every desire on your health wishlist.

A Pocket Guide to My Most Popular Programs

I have many different programs. For those wondering where to start, here's what I do with my clients: For people who have stopped being able to lose weight, who find it easier to gain than to lose, or who can't get their stalled metabolism moving again, I start with my flagship program, the Fast Metabolism Diet (we call it FMD). When my clients come to me with the complaint that their body shape or structure has changed, with fat pockets where they never had fat pockets before, or they say they just don't recognize themselves anymore, I start with Metabolism Revolution (we call it MR). When clients come to me totally tapped out and depleted, I put them on my 5-day or 10-day cleanse first. When people have longer-term goals, I like to rotate them through all the plans. For example, they might start with a 10-day cleanse, then do the Fast Metabolism Diet, then shift to Metabolism Revolution, then do a 5-day cleanse. This is a big-picture method for "confuse it to lose it" (the premise of the Fast Metabolism Diet, as you'll see below) while my clients get to eat amazing food all along the way. Here's more information on the primary plans I offer in my various books:

THE FAST METABOLISM DIET: A strategic way to use micronutrients and foods that have you cycling through different styles of eating to "confuse it to lose it." Just as you might cross-train your body to improve your athletic performance, cross-training your metabolism stimulates different burn, build, and restore mechanisms to maximize your efforts. I use this diet for my clients whose old tricks for weight loss don't work anymore. When you feel like your metabolism needs to be healed, when you feel like even *looking* at food makes you gain weight, or when you're under stress and your body won't let go of the fat because you're in crisis mode, this is the place to start. This diet is also good for hormone issues. Here's a summary of how it works:

- **Phase 1:** On Monday and Tuesday, you will unwind stress and calm the adrenals with lots of carbs and fruit.
- **Phase 2:** On Wednesday and Thursday, you will unlock fat stores and build muscle with lots of protein and veggies.
- **Phase 3:** On Friday through Sunday, you will unleash the burn by feeding your hormones to generate heat with moderate carbs, moderate protein, and lots of healthy fats and oils.

METABOLISM REVOLUTION: The Metabolism Revolution diet strategically manipulates macronutrients to speed the body's metabolic rate in order to provoke rapid weight loss, fat burning, muscle building, better skin, and boosted energy levels, and to reset your metabolism. This diet is best if you feel like your physical structure has changed and you don't recognize your body in the mirror anymore. It's also a good diet for those with high blood pressure. Each week is split into two parts of either three or four days each, with one style of eating for the first half and a different style of eating for the second half.

- **Part 1:** This part of the plan favors stress-reducing, energizing healthy carbs.
- **Part 2:** This part of the plan favors healing, building, sustaining protein.

5- AND 10-DAY FAST METABOLISM CLEANSES: These plans consist of my specially formulated whole-food powder and targeted nutrition programs designed to restore your natural detoxification system, returning your body to a healthy state so it can recover and function more efficiently. The 5-day cleanse is an intense way to clear your system of all the bad stuff that has made its way into your diet, pantry, and life. The 10-day cleanse is a life-changing way to kick-start rapid weight loss. It also cleanses your palate and hypernourishes with micronutrients and delicious food a body that has been tapped out, stressed out, or maxed out. You will cycle between whole-food meals and whole-food shakes to provoke a change in your metabolism.

THE BURN: The Burn is three unique nutrition plans that provoke microrepair in the metabolism to help break through weight loss plateaus caused by inflammation, digestion issues, or hormonal imbalances, in 3-, 5-, and 10-day plans.

- **I-Burn:** This 3-day plan flushes out excess water, reduces swelling, and takes down inflammation. You'll look like you lost a ton of weight in just three days, and roll right past any weight loss plateaus.
- **D-Burn:** This 5-day plan targets digestion, banishing belly bloat for a flat stomach and that high-energy good feeling you get when your digestion is running smoothly. If digestion has been impeding your weight loss, the D-Burn is your remedy.
- **H-Burn:** This 10-day plan tackles stubborn hormone-based weight loss resistance by flooding the body with micronutrients that restore hormone health so your body can relax and finally let go of the weight it has been holding on to.

FAST METABOLISM FOOD RX: Remember, Eating + Metabolism = Health. Health dysfunction is a metabolic adaptation, so correcting the metabolic pathways involved in different health issues can help to resolve those issues. This plan includes seven distinct eating programs to microfocus on the results of a dysfunctional metabolism:

- **Rx GI Dysfunction:** This plan focuses on what you absorb. It addresses GI dysfunctions like IBS, gas and bloating, acid reflux, and more, adjusting your gut function and microbiome health with targeted nutrition.

- **Rx Fatigue:** Address fatigue, lethargy, and exhaustion by removing what is blocking energy creation in your body and repairing the damage that stress, overexertion, disease, trauma, or environmental insult or injury has caused.
- **Rx Hormonal Imbalance:** When hormone production, metabolism, or absorption stop working the way they should, the result can be weight gain, muscle and collagen loss, thinning hair, PMS symptoms, thyroid dysregulation, hot flashes, and belly fat. This food prescription helps to restore hormonal balance.
- **Rx Impaired Cholesterol Metabolism:** Your ability to metabolize cholesterol directly impacts your hormonal function and brain chemistry. This plan helps to improve and regulate lipid metabolism by focusing on the liver, where cholesterol metabolism happens.
- **Rx Mood and Cognitive Challenges:** Mood changes and cognitive challenges like brain fog are often directly linked to diet, and a diet prescription can help stabilize these frustrating and potentially frightening issues.
- **Rx Impaired Sugar Metabolism:** The body uses sugar to create energy and build structures—and you only get it from food, including fresh fruits, veggies, and complex carbohydrates. If you can't metabolize sugar, you will experience blood sugar and insulin instability, which could result in metabolic syndrome, pre-diabetes, or diabetes. This plan can help

repair the pathways that facilitate sugar metabolism.
- **Rx Immune Dysregulation:** Autoimmune diseases like Hashimoto's disease, celiac disease, lupus, arthritis, multiple sclerosis, and many others can disrupt life and destroy function. This food prescription is powerful medicine to nurture the pathways that regulate the immune system.

WEEKEND WARRIOR: An intensive 2-day plan to flush out toxins and take down bloat and puffiness *fast*.

3-DAY SOUP CLEANSE: A 3-day plan featuring three powerful soups you get to enjoy five times per day to flood the body with nutrients, optimize the body's natural elimination process, nurture the liver, and stimulate the hormones that encourage satiety.

14-DAY PAIN AND INFLAMMATION PROTOCOL: Acute or chronic pain can be a symptom of inflammation, which can cause many different metabolic pathways to become stagnant or even create disease. This 14-day plan uses food-based shakes and strategic foods to help unlock pathways inhibited by inflammation.

FAST METABOLISM 4 LIFE: A comprehensive, modifiable nutrition program that continues to nurture and stoke the metabolism through the power of food. Many people use this for maintenance after they have achieved the reversal of metabolic dysfunction. Others adopt it as a basic strategy for healthy living.

PLAN-SWAPPING IN PRACTICE

It always impresses me how the members of our Fast Metabolism community decide to swap and hop and weave the different programs into their lives—especially when I see their amazing results. One member of our community, Margaret, is a great example of someone who uses all the programs for maximum benefit. Here's what she wrote to us recently:

" For me, Haylie's programs have been the way I address all the stages and events of my life. I first discovered the Fast Metabolism Diet after finding out my cholesterol was 206 and my triglycerides were 104. I also thought I could stand to lose a few pounds. On the Fast Metabolism Diet, I got my cholesterol down to 176 and my triglycerides down to 31! Awesome numbers. I also lost 5 pounds, which was great, but my doctor was most impressed with my improved test results. But then I asked myself: If food could do that for me, what else could it do? I have always been prone to digestive issues, so next I tried the D-Burn from Haylie's book *The Burn*. I couldn't believe how quickly my reflux and constipation resolved. I felt so good! But I didn't want to slip back into my old habits, and I also wanted to lose a few more pounds. That's when *Metabolism Revolution* came out. I took the tests and discovered that I needed Meal Map A, and after fourteen days on that program, I was down another 10 pounds and felt better than I had in years. Now I generally follow the maintenance program, Fast Metabolism 4 Life, but whenever I have an event coming up or swimsuit season looms, I do one of the 10-day Fast Metabolism Cleanse programs. I love having all these tools at my disposal. Haylie has a lifestyle for every need, and I plan to stick with her for life! What Haylie says really works. "

Now that you've got the big picture, let's get into your kitchen and start making some changes, so you will be fully prepared to start cooking.

HOW TO USE
THIS COOKBOOK

n order for you to get the most out of this cookbook, I first want you to get set up with some nuts and bolts. I'm going to show you:

- How to set up your kitchen, including how to keep your pantry and refrigerator clean, functional, and ready to cook.
- A comprehensive list of what to keep in your pantry so you have everything you need to make all the recipes in this book.
- A list of what should—and shouldn't—be in your refrigerator and freezer.
- My favorite go-to kitchen tools that I use over and over again and can't live without.
- How to navigate the Master Metabolism Food List and how to swap ingredients in recipes using this list if you cannot have an ingredient based on your preferences, allergies, nutritional needs, or philosophical/spiritual beliefs.
- The Master Metabolism Food List itself—eat from this list most of the time to keep your metabolism stoked every day.
- How to figure out servings and portion sizes and how to divide recipes for multiple people or for freezing.
- How to make a super-simple meal map to get you organized for the week.
- How to make multiple batches of the recipes, including an easy plan for cooking a full 30 days of meals ahead of time so they are ready to go right from your freezer. It's a great solution for when you have a lot going on and know you won't have time to cook.
- The icing on the cake (no pun intended): how to modify and use each and every one of the recipes in this book on any one of my therapeutic plans, including the Fast Metabolism Diet, The Burn, Fast Metabolism Food Rx, Fast Metabolism Revolution, and Fast Metabolism 4 Life. If you are on one of my programs, this cookbook will greatly expand your options and refresh your experience with new, exciting ways to use food strategically to reach your goals.

Let's dive right in!

How to Set Up Your Kitchen

First, let's talk about my favorite room in my house (or any house). Kitchens are highly personal, and how they are designed will ideally reflect the person who uses them. But even if you aren't about to remodel your kitchen, there are many ways you can personalize it to match the way you use it and to make it more comfortable, comforting, and meaningful for you. Having recently designed my own kitchen when I was moving into a new house, I've discovered a few strategies that are highly effective for creating a usable kitchen that will quickly become the center of your home. Here are some features in mine:

- A central gathering area. We put in a large island with space for cooking on one side and room for family members and friends to sit, snack, do homework, play games, or just relax, talk, and laugh on the other side. When I'm cooking, I can be right in the center of the action. Of course, if you like to cook in private or don't want people getting in the way, you may prefer that people gather in the dining room or a separate part of the kitchen, leaving your cooking space to yourself.
- Plenty of cutting boards. Whether they are built in or just easily accessible, cutting boards make it fast and easy to cut up veggies or fruit—and I always want you to eat more veggies!
- Drawers and pull-out cabinet shelves. These make it easy to find things, even when they are in the back of your cabinet.
- More refrigerator and freezer space than pantry space. People often ask me why I have one large and three additional small refrigerators in my kitchen. I need the space! Most of the food you eat should be fresh, so make plenty of room. Your crisper isn't enough space for the bounty of vegetables and fruits you're going to bring into your life. It can also be helpful to organize your refrigerator and freezer spaces with baskets, trays, boxes, or other organizing containers to maximize the space. You might consider putting a mini fridge or freezer in your garage or on the back porch (if you live in a temperate climate). The more space you have, the better.

- Accessible, easy-to-view spice racks. I depend on herbs and spices to add excitement to food, so I use them constantly. I hope you will, too—and making seasonings accessible can help inspire you to use them liberally. I built spice racks on both sides of my stove so I can easily grab any herb or spice I need. But you don't have to build them in. There are many handy spice racks and lazy susans that can hold your spices, in or out of cabinets. You can also find DIY spice rack designs online or have them retrofitted into your current cabinets. I've also seen spice racks that can hang over a door and magnetic spice racks you can put right on your refrigerator.

- A no-cleaning-chemicals configuration. When we were putting in my kitchen sink, I decided to put my drain on the right side of a double sink instead of on the left. This freed up that dead space under my sink, and that is where I keep my kitchen trash. I've seen people with picture-perfect, pristine, organized refrigerators, but then I see under the sink. It's often dirty, cluttered, and worst of all, full of cleaning products containing chemical obesogens. Remember that toxins you put on your countertops and other surfaces can transfer to your food and end up stored in your fat cells. Be aware that 60 percent of what comes into contact with your skin gets absorbed, and smelling something is also a mode of consumption (also keep this in mind with synthetic air fresheners and scented candles). So, if you touch a cleaner or smell a cleaner, you're consuming that cleaner. You may be thinking, "What's under my sink is under my sink. It's not like I'm adding it to my salad dressing," but you don't need to put something in your mouth to be exposed to it. Stick with all-natural cleaners, and—for the sake of organization and a sense of safety and purity—keep cleaners out of your kitchen. A good rule of thumb is that your kitchen should contain only things that go in your mouth or help get things into your mouth. A place for everything, and everything in its place.

Spice Rack Basics

Whether you're creating a new spice rack or just refreshing your old one, know that herbs and spices can expire and lose potency. Go through your spices and throw away any that are more than a year old, then restock with new containers of herbs and spices you will actually use regularly.

This is a list of all the herbs and spices you will need to make every recipe in this book. It's a good place to start. You can always expand your spice repertoire as you become more confident in the kitchen and find yourself ready to experiment with more flavors.

HERBS (DRIED)

- Basil
- Bay leaves
- Cilantro
- Dill weed
- Italian seasoning
- Marjoram
- Mint
- Oregano (any type)
- Parsley
- Rosemary
- Sage
- Savory
- Tarragon
- Thyme

SPICES (DRIED, WHOLE, GROUND, OR FRESHLY GRATED)

- Black pepper
- Cardamom
- Cayenne pepper
- Chili powder
- Chipotle powder
- Cinnamon
- Cloves
- Coriander
- Cumin
- Curry powder
- Fenugreek
- Five-spice powder (sometimes called Chinese five-spice, organic only)
- Garlic powder
- Ginger
- Mustard (dried)
- Nutmeg
- Onion powder
- Paprika (sweet, Hungarian, and smoked)
- Red pepper flakes
- Turmeric

EXTRACTS (REAL OR PURE, NOT ARTIFICIAL OR IMITATION)

- Mint
- Vanilla

Your Pantry

Hear ye, hear ye: *It is time to gut your kitchen!* I don't mean you have to tear out the drywall. But the first step in setting up a dream pantry is to get rid of all the packaged, processed food that lives there now. You don't need it, and your metabolism will suffer if you eat it. While I mostly want to eat fresh food, the pantry can be a place for basic whole-food staples. If you peeked into my pantry, you wouldn't see much in the way of packages. Instead, I fill up Mason jars with raw nuts, chia seeds, flaxseeds, brown rice, oats, and quinoa. Mason jars keep your dry goods fresh, they look beautiful, and it's easy to see what's in them. I put my pasta in those tall, clear pasta containers with sealed lids. I cut out the label on the package and tape it to the front. I have cans of beans and tomatoes, olive oil and safflower oil, some very basic unopened condiments (like no-sugar-added ketchup and mustard), and a few baking essentials like baking soda, almond flour, and arrowroot powder.

I suggest first taking everything out of your pantry, cleaning the pantry shelves, then putting back only items from the following list. These are the only things that should be in your pantry. Get rid of the packages, cereal boxes, wrapped bars, and snack packets, the dinner-in-a-box flavored rice and pasta mixes and sauces, the cans of salty soup, and anything else with a long ingredients list. For everything else, open those bags and boxes of grains, nuts, and seeds, and put them in Mason jars or other sealable storage containers, clearly labeled and easy to see. When foods are packaged in paper or cardboard, it can be harder to reseal them when you use some of the product. Organic and preservative-free foods in particular have a shorter shelf life, so sealing them can help you get the maximum freshness time. Also, it's easier for little bugs to get into your grains, nuts, and seeds if they're stored in boxes and bags. Organic food with no preservatives and pesticides is especially attractive to those little bugs—it's good food for them—so sealing up foods like rice, oats, barley, almonds, and pumpkin seeds can keep out the critters. A friend once told me that she leaves her packages of white rice open and she doesn't get bugs. I told her to try that with organic brown rice and see what happens! (Note that for even longer preservation, you may want to keep grains, nuts, and seeds in your freezer.)

With these basics in your pantry, you will never be without something wholesome and real to eat.

Pantry List

Baking powder

Baking soda

Beans/legumes
(canned or dried)
- Black beans
- Chickpeas/garbanzo beans
- Lentils
- Pinto beans
- White beans

Broth (no sugar added only,
or make your own [see
page 274])
- Beef
- Chicken
- Vegetable

Cacao (raw)
- Cacao nibs
- Cacao powder

Coconut
- Coconut flakes (unsweetened)
- Coconut water (unsweetened)

Condiments (store
in the refrigerator after
opening)
- Hot sauce (no additives,
  such as Frank's RedHot or
  Tabasco)
- Ketchup (no sugar added,
  or make your own
  [see page 267])

- Mustard, especially Dijon
  (no sugar added)
- Salsa (or make your own
  [see page 267])

Flavorings, natural:
- Liquid smoke
- Nutritional yeast
- Red chile paste

Flours from any allowed
ingredients, including:
- Almond flour
- Amaranth flour
- Brown rice flour
- Cassava flour
- Chickpea flour (aka besan or
  garbanzo bean flour)
- Coconut flour
- Oat flour
- Spelt flour

Fruit, dried:
- Prunes only

Grains
- Brown rice, brown rice pasta,
  puffed brown rice, brown rice
  milk (unsweetened)
- Oats (old-fashioned or rolled,
  steel-cut, or quick-cooking)
- Quinoa (any color), puffed
  quinoa
- Spelt
- Sprouted grain bread, buns,
  tortillas

Mayonnaise (refrigerate
after opening)

- Avocado oil mayo
- Safflower oil mayo

Milks (non-dairy only,
unsweetened only, in pure
form) from any allowed
ingredients, including:

- Almond milk
- Brown rice milk
- Cashew milk
- Coconut milk (full-fat,
  canned)
- Coconut milk (boxed,
  unsweetened)
- Hemp milk
- Macadamia milk
- Oat milk
- Pea milk (from chickpeas, yel-
  low peas, or lentils, not green
  peas)
- Quinoa milk
- Combinations of the above
  types, such as coconut-
  almond milk

Nuts

- Almonds, almond butter,
  almond flour
- Cashews, cashew butter
- Pecans
- Pine nuts
- Walnuts

Oils

- Coconut oil
- Grapeseed oil

- Olive oil
- Safflower oil
- Sesame oil

Sea salt

Seeds

- Black and white
  sesame seeds
- Chia seeds
- Flaxseed (whole
  or ground)
- Pumpkin seeds (pepitas,
  hulled, raw)
- Sunflower seeds (hulled)

Soy sauce replacements

- Coconut aminos
- Liquid aminos
- Tamari

Sweeteners (always
optional, 100% pure,
no additives)

- Monk fruit (lo han)
- Stevia
- Xylitol

Thickeners

- Agar-agar
- Arrowroot powder

Vinegars

- Apple cider vinegar
- Balsamic vinegar
- Red wine vinegar
- Rice vinegar (unseasoned/
  unsweetened only)
- White wine vinegar

Refrigerator

Just as we began in the pantry, the first step toward refrigerator bliss is to take out the trash. Empty your refrigerator and get rid of those condiments that are decades old (everybody's got them), the old grape jelly, the hardened peanut butter, the little bits of leftovers pushed to the back, the rotting produce. Give everything a good cleaning, then vow that your refrigerator is for real food only. That means:

- Fresh vegetables
- Fresh herbs
- Fresh fruit
- Meat

- Seafood
- Nut/seed/grain milk
- Opened containers of no-sugar-added condiments (like mayo, ketchup, and mustard)

Fresh Produce Tips

We've all been there: Those beautiful tomatoes, those luscious strawberries, that crisp lettuce gets wilted, old, even slimy before you get a chance to eat it. What a waste! To avoid losing your produce, here are some of my favorite tips:

- When you store your salad greens and fresh herbs, put a small amount of air in your sealed bag along with a paper towel to absorb moisture.
- All veggies and fruits last longer if you keep the stems on. That goes for apples, avocados, carrots, beets, radishes, and tomatoes. When choosing your produce, look for veggies and fruits with the stems

or greenery attached for maximum storage time.

- Not all veggies and fruits go in the refrigerator. Leave tomatoes, bananas, unripe peaches and pears, and avocados on the counter (but away from the heat of the stove). Baskets and bowls are nice for holding these.
- Potatoes and onions will last longer if you keep them in a cool, dark place, such as in a wire or mesh basket or bag in a cabinet. Store them apart, however, as they both release compounds that can cause the other to rot faster.

Freezer

This is primarily the place to organize all the food you have made ahead. (You'll read more about how to do this starting on page 66.) Personally, I'm obsessed with making big batches and freezing meals. I also love freezer containers that stack and waste as little space as possible. I write with crayon on my freezer containers, labeling and dating everything on the front so I can quickly see what's in those containers without pulling them all out. When I make a big batch of White Chicken Chili (page 191), I let it cool off, then store it in labeled zip-top freezer bags stacked in shoebox-size containers, also labeled. It's one of my favorite freezer recipes. Another favorite for the freezer is Baked Buffalo Wings (page 253). These freeze surprisingly well, and I always have some ready for an anytime snack or for when a spontaneous party breaks out and I want to serve something I know I can eat and that everyone else will love, too.

To take maximum advantage of your freezer, clean it out and get rid of all the old freezer-burned packaged food you keep thinking you might eat it someday but know you really won't, so you have room for all the great meals and snacks you're going to make from this book. My freezer mantra is: Get rid of all your packaged food and replace it with food *you* have packaged.

I also keep two bags in my freezer for produce that is getting a little wilted—one for fruit that's almost too ripe, which I can use in smoothies, and one for vegetables that are just starting to wilt, which I can use to make broth. When I'm ready to make that smoothie—maybe the Strawberry Rhubarb Pie Smoothie (page 85)—or broth—like Basic Vegetable Broth (page 274)—I just take out the appropriate bag and empty it into the blender or the stockpot.

On the Counter

Sometimes I keep a bowl of fruit on my counter, but most of the time, I keep fruit in tiered hanging baskets to keep different kinds separate—especially apples and oranges. Oranges contain bioflavonoids that can soften apples, and since I like my apples crisp, I keep them separated. As an added bonus, keeping fruit in plain sight, no matter how you store it, can encourage you and your family to choose it for a snack rather than something packaged. The easier something is to grab, the more likely someone will grab it.

BANANAS: A RIPENING TOOL

I don't usually eat bananas because they're not the best fruit for boosting the metabolism, but my daughter loves them, so I always have them in my house. For me, they are a ripening tool. Bananas release ethylene gas, which is the same gas commercial farmers use to ripen produce that they have picked early. If you store other produce, like avocados, pears, or apples, with your bananas, it will ripen fast. You can use this to your advantage. If your avocado is *almost* ripe and you want to use it for dinner tonight, or you want to ripen up those tomatoes quickly, take the stems off and put the tomatoes in a bag with some bananas. (For rock-hard avocados and green tomatoes, ripening by banana can take a few days.) But if you want your pears to last more than a couple of days, keep them away from the bananas!

My Go-To Kitchen Supplies

Honestly, I don't use that many different kitchen tools. I rely on a few basics that can handle any job in this book and most other cooking tasks. These are my go-tos that I use all the time:

- Baking pan, 8- or 9-inch square—the perfect size for treats like Baked Carrot Cake Oatmeal (page 93).
- Baking sheet with a rim (sometimes it's nice to have two). These are especially good for saucy roly-poly foods, like Baked Buffalo Wings (page 253) or Three-Way Roasted Chickpeas (page 247).
- Blender, a high-quality one that can handle tough jobs. I use mine frequently, especially for breakfast when I might want a Spa Smoothie (page 85) or Mint Chocolate Chip Smoothie Bowl (page 90).

- Broiling pan, which I use whenever I don't want to fire up the grill, for savory recipes like Steak Breakfast Fajitas (page 109) or Sweet Potato Turkey Burger Sliders (page 162).
- Casserole dish with a lid, which is perfect for baking Easy Turkey Noodle Casserole (page 196) or Taco Pasta Casserole (page 207).
- Chef's knife. A good-quality one that feels right in your hand will make cutting easier. Keep it sharp—you'll be doing a lot of chopping, slicing, and mincing.
- Cutting boards, the more the better. I prefer wooden and bamboo types. A lot of plastic ones have antibacterial chemicals added to them that can adulterate your incredibly valuable and precious food.
- Food processor, for chopping up Fire-Roasted Salsa (page 267) and creating smooth, creamy condiments like Coconut Sour Cream (page 263) and Cashew Sour Cream (page 263).
- Freezer storage containers. Get stackable ones that fit into the corners of your freezer, with a spot to affix labels.
- Mason jars for pantry storage. These are perfect for your grains, nuts, and seeds.
- Muffin tins. I have a standard one and a mini one, which I use for meals such as Breakfast Muffin Tin Meat Loaf (page 125) or Muffin Tin Chicken Potpies (page 186).
- Parchment paper, for all oil-free and nonstick uses. Parchment paper is great for lining baking pans or even skillets, or for recipes like Crispy Quinoa Chia Bars (page 88) or the Chef's Salad Parchment Wrap (page 141).
- Saucepans, one medium and one large, with lids. I use mine every day for everything from actual sauces to warming up soups and boiling eggs.
- Silicone-tipped tongs. I use these to toss Cinnamon Jicama Fries (page 261), pull tortilla bowls out of the oven for a Taco Lime Shrimp Salad (page 144), and flip turkey bacon.
- Skillet, high-quality with a lid and high sides so you can also stir-fry in it. I like cast iron, but a heavy-bottomed, good-quality stainless-steel skillet is also a good choice. I use mine for almost every meal.
- Slow cooker, for those days when you want to come home to a hot meal that's ready to go, like Cashew Soup (page 136) or Slow Cooker Greek Drumsticks (page 195).
- Spiralizer. You don't *really* need this because you could cut any vegetable into noodle shapes by hand with a knife, but it's fun to use, and you can replace the pasta in any

recipe, from Spaghetti Bolognese (page 210) to Chicken Piccata (page 185), with spiralized zucchini, sweet potatoes, or broccoli stems.

- Stockpot with a lid, for making Basic Vegetable Broth (page 274) or cooking large amounts of any soup, stew, or casserole.
- Vegetable peeler, for cleaning up those carrots and peeling sweet potatoes.

About the Recipes

I had several goals when I was creating the recipes in this book. One was to make every recipe well balanced, with a diversity of macronutrients (protein, carbohydrates, fat) and micronutrients (vitamins, minerals, and phytochemicals from plant foods). Another was to make the recipes taste amazing. My favorite way to do this is to incorporate herbs and spices and a lot of vegetables—each of these has enzymes that help with digestion and micronutrient extraction, and also adds flavors, textures, and more interest to every recipe.

But you don't need to overdo it, especially where the herbs and spices are concerned. Not everyone likes strong-tasting food. These recipes are designed for the more sensitive tongue, but I encourage you to spice them up whenever you can. For example, when I make Beef Lo Mein (page 209), I double the amount of red chile paste . . . but I keep a large glass of lemon water close at hand! (Lemon can help quench the burn.) Add spices a little at a time until you get the taste you like—you can always spice up, but you can't spice down.

I also encourage your creativity. I'm not a cook who typically measures or weighs my ingredients. I like to wing it and see what happens. You can always add more or fewer spices than I call for. You can add more or different vegetables. When I experiment, it doesn't always work out the way I imagined. Sometimes I need to try a few different versions to find the flavors I want, but that's all part of the fun and the learning process. It's what keeps me coming back to the kitchen. Cooking can be an endless opportunity to exercise your curiosity and your sense of adventure. These recipes are just a road map, and you can always take a detour.

Servings and Portion Sizes

People often get confused about what constitutes a portion or a serving size. I find that in many cases, it's not just difficult but inaccurate to designate an exact portion size like "1 cup" or "4 ounces," because the ingredients people use vary and the methods and cooking times can also influence volume. That's why I prefer that you designate your portion sizes based on how many people each recipe serves. Every recipe tells you at the top how many servings are in that recipe. If a recipe serves four, then a portion is simply one-quarter of the full recipe. Here are some ways to serve everyone the correct portion:

- You can put the whole thing in a measuring cup. If you're making the Poblano Pork Chili Verde in the Skillet (page 215), which serves eight, and your finished dish fills up an 8-cup measuring bowl, you know that each serving is 1 cup. You can divide the rice among eight bowls and put 1 cup of the chili verde in each.
- You can divide a finished recipe among serving plates and storage containers. For example, let's say you're making Slow Cooker Hungarian Goulash (page 212). That recipe serves eight. Maybe you're serving four people for dinner that night, and you want to pack up four additional servings for future lunches or quick din-

ners. When you're ready to serve the goulash, set out four individual serving plates and four freezer containers, then ladle the goulash evenly among the plates and containers, one ladle at a time. When the slow cooker is empty, each plate and each storage container will contain one portion.

- If your recipe is something you can cut into pieces, like the Oven-Baked Stuffed Pork Roast (page 216), slice or cut the portions evenly.
- For a recipe like the Grilled Fish Tostadas (page 224) that serves four and makes eight tostadas, you can easily see that each portion includes two tostadas.
- For any recipe in this book, if you need to serve more people than the indicated number of servings, you can double or triple the ingredients. For example, if you're making Spaghetti Squash Shrimp and Artichoke Alfredo (page 219), which serves four, but you want to serve a group of eight people, you could double all the ingredients.

I don't want you to worry about measuring every drop or piece of food exactly. I've designed these recipes so that serving yourself approximately one-quarter of a recipe that serves four people total is fine.

About the Master Metabolism Food List

I recommend you eat from this list of all the metabolism-boosting foods most of the time. Even without looking at a single recipe, you could live off the foods on this list and know you are boosting your metabolism with nutrient-rich whole foods. The Master Metabolism Food List is divided by category: Vegetables, Fruits, Proteins (Animal and Vegetable), Seafood, Grains, Healthy Fats, and Miscellaneous (condiments, flavorings, thickeners, etc.). Each category specifies what form to choose. For example, the Fruits list specifies "fresh or frozen only." I recommend avoiding canned fruit because the cooking and canning process typically increases its glycemic load.

Each item on the list also includes guidance for portion sizes. For example, an avocado portion is half an avocado; a rice portion is 1 cup cooked; and a portion of fish is 6 ounces, weighed before cooking. Note that the portion sizes are suggestions and represent nice, healthy amounts of food for the average person. If you need more or less, that's generally fine. What's most important is the quality and wholeness of the foods you're eating. If you are (or have been) on any of my plans, you may have noticed that different plans have variable portion sizes based on the weight loss and other health goals of that particular plan. In this cookbook, the portion strategy is simple: to speed up the metabolism. Remember that eating is the key, so eat enough for your needs—especially vegetables. This is why I say "at least 2 cups" for vegetables. All my plans use vegetables therapeutically, and nearly all vegetables are listed with unlimited portions. Think of vegetables as kindling for your metabolic fire. Not getting enough can inhibit your efforts to kick-start your metabolism.

This list is also your guide to adapting the recipes according to your needs. Do you need to change an ingredient? No problem. Whether it's for convenience, cost, seasonality, availability, medical reasons, or your preference, you can always swap an undesired ingredient for something you love. Just flip over to the Master Metabolism Food List, go to that ingredient's category (for example, beef is under "Proteins," pineapples are under "Fruits"), and scroll down the list. You can substitute any ingredient for any other ingredient in the same category. For example, you could substitute broccoli for green beans, brown rice for barley, cilantro for parsley, chicken for pork, pineapple for mango. A Cherry Almond Smoothie Bowl (page 87) could become a blackberry almond smoothie bowl by substituting blackberries for the cherries. The brown rice vermicelli in your Chicken Piccata (page 185) could be replaced by spiralized zucchini noodles. The cilantro-lime vinaigrette on your Southwest Breakfast Salad (page 104) could be swapped out for basil-lime vinaigrette or dill-lemon vinaigrette.

This substitution strategy expands the recipes in this cookbook almost infinitely. You will never run out of variations if you make good use of this Master Metabolism Food List, which contains all the foods that fuel your metabolism and none that slow it down. If you stick to this list whenever you eat and vary the foods you eat as much as possible, you will be giving your body the tools it needs to thrive, lose weight, and get optimally healthy.

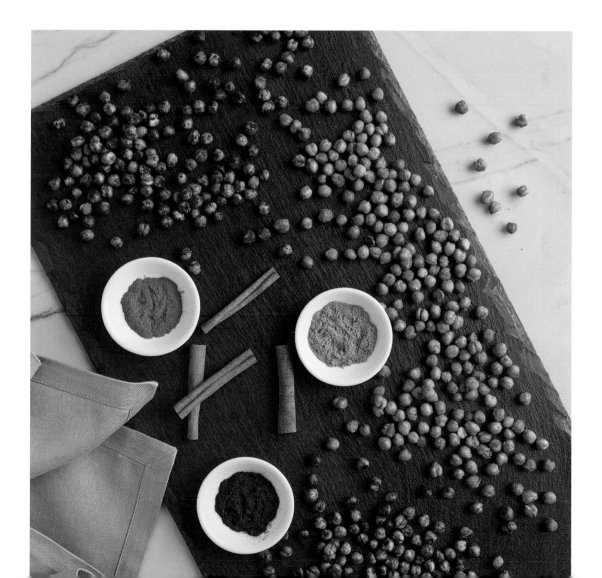

MASTER METABOLISM FOOD LIST

VEGETABLES

Portion: Minimum 2 cups raw

- Artichokes
- Asparagus
- Bamboo shoots
- Beans: green, yellow (wax), French (haricots verts), string
- Beets, all
- Broccoli/Broccolini
- Brussels sprouts
- Cabbage, all types (including bok choy and fermented/cultured cabbage such as sauerkraut and kimchi)
- Cactus
- Carrots
- Cauliflower
- Celery
- Cucumbers, all types
- Cultured/fermented veggies, all types
- Eggplant
- Endive (including chicory and radicchio)
- Fennel
- Hearts of palm
- Jicama
- Kohlrabi
- Leafy greens, all types (including spinach, kale, collards, dandelion greens, etc., and all lettuce except iceberg)
- Mushrooms, all types
- Okra
- Onions, all (including scallions, leeks, and shallots)
- Parsnips
- Peas: snap, snow (not green peas)
- Peppers, all
- Pumpkin
- Radishes (including daikon)
- Rhubarb
- Rutabaga
- Sea vegetables and seaweeds: dulse, hijiki, kelp, kombu, nori
- Spirulina
- Sprouts, all
- Squash, all
- Sweet potatoes, all
- Tomatillos
- Tomatoes, all
- Turnips
- Yams
- Zucchini

FRUITS
(FRESH OR FROZEN ONLY)

Portion: 1 cup raw or frozen

- Apples, all
- Apricots, all

- Bananas (in moderation)
- Berries, all
- Cherimoya
- Cherries
- Clementines
- Dates (fresh only, in moderation)
- Figs (fresh only)
- Grapefruit
- Guavas
- Honeydew melon
- Kiwi
- Kumquats
- Lemons
- Limes
- Loquats
- Mangoes
- Melons, all
- Nectarines
- Oranges
- Papaya
- Peaches
- Pears, all
- Persimmons
- Pineapple
- Plums
- Pluots
- Pomegranates
- Prickly pears
- Prunes (this is the only allowed dried fruit)
- Tangerines

PROTEINS (ANIMAL AND VEGETABLE)

Portion size: 4 ounces raw for animal protein, tempeh, and tofu; ½ cup cooked for beans/legumes; 2 large eggs/4 egg whites

- Beans/legumes, all except peanuts and green peas (includes lentils, black beans, chickpeas, lima beans, etc.)
- Beef, lean cuts only
- Buffalo
- Chicken, all
- Cornish game hen
- Deli meats: chicken, roast beef, turkey (nitrate-free, no sugar added)
- Eggs, all
- Gelatin (from grass-fed beef only)
- Jerky, all (nitrate-free, no sugar added)
- Lamb, lean cuts only
- Organ meats, all
- Pork, lean cuts only
- Rabbit
- Sausages, nitrate-free, no sugar added: turkey, chicken
- Turkey, all, including nitrate-free, no-sugar-added turkey bacon
- Wild game, all

SEAFOOD

Portion size: 6 ounces raw

- Calamari
- Caviar
- Clams
- Crab
- Crawfish
- Fish, wild-caught, any type
- Lobster
- Mussels
- Oysters
- Scallops
- Shrimp

GRAINS

Portion: 1 cup cooked, 1 slice bread, 1 (8-ounce) tortilla, 1 ounce crackers, ½ cup baking mix

Note: Many products are made with the following grains, including pasta, bread, tortillas, milk, etc. These are all acceptable unless they contain ingredients not found on this master foods list. Also note that all sprouted grains are okay.

- Amaranth
- Barley
- Buckwheat
- Einkorn
- Farro
- Fast Metabolism Baking Mix
- Freekeh
- Kamut
- Millet
- Oats
- Quinoa
- Rice: brown, black, purple, red, wild
- Rye (any rye product must be 100% rye)
- Sorghum
- Spelt
- Sprouted wheat
- Tapioca
- Teff

HEALTHY FATS

Portion: See each ingredient

Note: Many products are made with the nuts and seeds on this list, including bread, butter, cheese, milk, tortillas, yogurt, etc. These are all acceptable unless they contain ingredients not found on this master foods list. Note that nuts, seeds, and nut and seed butters should *always be raw,* with no additives or sweetener.

- Avocado: ½
- Coconut: raw meat, butter, cream, milk (no sugar): ¼ cup
- Hummus: ⅓ cup
- Mayonnaise (made with any oil from this list): 2 to 4 tablespoons
- Oils: avocado, coconut, grapeseed, olive, safflower, sesame, sunflower, walnut: 2 to 4 tablespoons

- Olives: 8 to 10
- Nut and seed butters (raw only): 2 tablespoons
- Nuts and seeds, all (raw only): ¼ cup
- Tahini (sesame seed butter): 2 tablespoons

MISCELLANEOUS (CONDIMENTS, FLAVORINGS, THICKENERS, ETC.)

- Birch xylitol
- Brewer's yeast
- Broth/stock, homemade or natural, no sugar added: beef, chicken, turkey, vegetable
- Cacao, raw
- Capers
- Carob
- Coconut water, unsweetened
- Coffee substitutes: Dandy Blend, Pero
- Extracts/flavorings, all (pure only, no sugar added, no alcohol, no artificial coloring)
- Fast Metabolism Quick & Easy Dessert and Snack Mix
- Garlic
- Ginger

- Herbal tea (caffeine-free)
- Herbs and spices, dried or fresh, all
- Horseradish
- Hot sauce (containing vinegar, peppers, and seasonings only)
- Ketchup (no sugar or corn syrup added)
- Liquid aminos or coconut aminos
- Monk fruit extract (pure only, no additives)
- Mustard, all (no sugar added)
- Nutritional yeast
- Pickles (no sugar added)
- Psyllium husk
- Salsa (including fermented)
- Sea salt
- Shirataki noodles
- Stevia (pure only, no additives)
- Tamari
- Thickeners: agar-agar, arrowroot powder, guar gum, xanthan gum
- Vinegars, all (pure, no additives)
- Water chestnuts
- Wheatgrass juice (2 to 4 ounces)

Meal Planning

Now that you have your Master Metabolism Food List, it's time to talk about meal planning. The more you plan, the easier it will be to stay on track and keep your diet full of real food without resorting to junk, drive-throughs, or delivery. Meal planning also makes it easier to mix up your recipes for more variety. In every one of my programs, I teach people how to make meal maps that keep them on track and give them a calm sense of organization and intention, but you don't have to be on one of my programs to take advantage of meal mapping.

This cookbook contains thirty days of recipes, organized by Breakfast, Lunch, Dinner, Snacks, and Desserts. With thirty breakfasts, thirty lunches, thirty dinners, five snacks, and five desserts, you could technically eat a different dish at every meal every day for a month before you had to have anything twice. But I know that's not how most people work, myself included. Everyone has a different style of cooking and different time constraints, so I designed this cookbook to be ultimately adaptable to you and your schedule.

You can plan out your meals one day at a time or, even better (especially for shopping purposes), a week at a time. Print out your blank meal map and fill it out before you do your weekly shopping trip. You can use the recipes in this book or any foods from the Master Metabolism Food List (page 58). Make a plan for every breakfast, lunch, dinner, and all the snacks you think you'll want. Fill out the shopping list with everything you'll need for the week that you don't already have in your (now perfectly organized!) pantry, refrigerator, or freezer.

A few things to think about as you map out your meals:

- I recommend having no dish more than three times per week (one of the strategies I outlined in chapter one) and no dish two days in a row. This will maximize the variety in your diet and give you the widest range of micronutrients. I know how easy it is to have leftovers from dinner the night before for lunch the next day, but I prefer freezing the leftovers to eat at least a few days later. If you want to change the outcome of your current health situation, you need to have control over what and how you eat. Food rotation is one fairly easy way to make a big impact on your health, due both to reducing overexposure to foods that may be causing reactions for you and in increasing micronutrient diversity. Don't hesitate to make food in large batches, label them, and put them in the freezer so you always have an abundance of grab-and-go food.

- Meal map with your calendar so you can factor in any events, meetings, parties, or holidays when you know you'll be eating out or anything else that might impact what you'll be eating.
- Any one meal can be swapped for another. You can always have breakfast for dinner, dinner for breakfast, dinner for lunch, or flip your snacks and meals to work better with your schedule.
- Don't forget all those handy meals you've packed away (or will soon pack away) in your freezer. Plan to use those on the days you know you'll be busy. You can keep most meals in the freezer in airtight freezer containers for 2 to 3 months. If you invest in a vacuum sealer, you can keep vacuum-sealed foods in a deep freezer for many months or even up to a year.

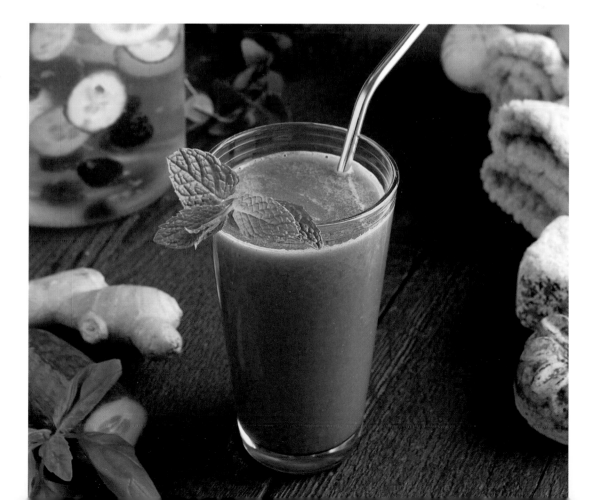

To see how this works, here's a meal map from one of my clients.

	Breakfast	Snack	Lunch	Snack	Dinner
Monday	Minty Melon Salad (page 101)	Almonds	Crunchy Broccoli Apple Chicken Salad (page 143)	Baked Buffalo Wings (page 253)	Parchment-Baked Salmon and Veggies (page 222)
Tuesday	Jicama Toast with Egg (page 113)	Chocolate-Orange Power Balls (page 250)	Beef Bulgogi Lettuce Cups (page 147)	Orange	Mediterranean Veggie Burgers with Aioli Slaw (page 232)
Wednesday	Baked Carrot Cake Oatmeal (page 93)	Apple	Business Lunch: Eating Out	Cinnamon Chickpeas (page 247)	Brazilian Fish Stew (page 230)
Thursday	Crispy Quinoa Chia Bars (page 88)	Baked Buffalo Wings (page 253)	Cashew Soup (page 136)	Spicy Salmon Jerky (page 248)	Korean BBQ Bowl with Jackfruit and Rhubarb Sauce (page 237)
Friday	Spa Smoothie (page 85)	Red Hot Chili Chickpeas (page 247)	Steak Stew (page 139)	Mango slices	Date Night: Eating Out
Saturday	Black- and Blueberry Quinoa Breakfast Salad (page 102)	Spicy Salmon Jerky (page 248)	Crustless Quiche (page 107) (*Note that she chose to have a breakfast recipe for lunch here*)	Grilled Mushroom Skewers with Balsamic Glaze (page 245)	Vegetarian Baked Lasagna (page 241)
Sunday	Steak Breakfast Fajitas (page 109)	Mango slices	Mushroom Soup (page 133)	Curry Chickpeas (page 247)	Slow Cooker Greek Drumsticks with Asparagus (page 195)

As she made this list, she also made her shopping list. Because she packed up and froze many of the extra portions for these meals, her following week was similar, but she didn't have to cook very much because she was eating fresh "fast food" from her freezer that she had prepared herself.

Now you try. Here's a blank meal map you can use to plan out your week, using the recipes in this book and your favorite foods from the Master Metabolism Food List (page 58). As you add each recipe, be sure to add what you don't already have on hand to your shopping list. If you plan and shop (and maybe even cook some things ahead—see page 66) on the weekend, you'll be ready to go for Monday. On page 66, there are lists for writing out all the food ingredients you'll need for your chosen recipes, along with a separate list for the items you already have, so when you're at the grocery store, you won't have to try to remember if you have any cumin or frozen cherries or enough brown rice left for the recipes you're making that week.

	Breakfast	Snack	Lunch	Snack	Dinner
Monday					
Tuesday					
Wednesday					
Thursday					
Friday					
Saturday					
Sunday					

Shopping List: Foods I Need	Foods I Need That I Already Have
_____	_____
_____	_____
_____	_____
_____	_____
_____	_____
_____	_____
_____	_____
_____	_____
_____	_____
_____	_____
_____	_____

Meal Planning—and Cooking— for a Month of "Fast Food"

As you know by now, I like to make big batches of food, doubling or tripling recipes, and freeze portions so I always have a meal ready to go in the freezer for those nights when I don't have time to cook. My community has gotten pretty savvy about doing this, too. They post pictures of their meals and how they've stored them, labeled according to their phases (if they are doing the Fast Metabolism Diet) or according to whatever plan they're doing. This can be you!

If you cook bigger batches and freeze them, you can pretty easily prepare, pack, label, and freeze an entire month's worth of meals at once, rotated so that you never repeat a meal too often. All you have to do is follow this plan. Just choose seven recipes and make enough of each to serve twelve people. This will feed you for twenty-eight full days! It's easier than you think. Here's how:

STEP ONE: Choose seven meals according to these criteria:

Recipe A: Dinner recipe.

Recipe B: Versatile recipe that you might have for breakfast, lunch, or dinner.

Recipe C: Breakfast recipe (such as oatmeal).

Recipe D: Recipe that could be lunch or dinner.

Recipe E: Recipe that could be breakfast or lunch.

Recipe F: Recipe that could be breakfast or lunch.

Recipe G: Recipe that could be lunch or dinner.

STEP TWO: Go grocery shopping to get everything you need to make all seven recipes in an amount that serves twelve. Also pick up the snacks you like from the Snack recipes starting on page 244.

STEP THREE: Make twelve portions of all seven meals. Pack them into freezer containers and label them with the recipe name and letter. Stack them in your freezer so it's easy to see the letter on each container.

STEP FOUR: Follow this schedule four times (for one person) or two times (for two people). Voilà—two to four weeks of wholesome real-food meals, no daily cooking!

30-Day Super-Simple Meal Plan

	Breakfast	**Snack**	**Lunch**	**Snack**	**Dinner**
Monday	C	Any snack	D	Any snack	A
Tuesday	E	Any snack	G	Any snack	B
Wednesday	C	Any snack	F	Any snack	D
Thursday	F	Any snack	B	Any snack	A
Friday	E	Any snack	G	Any snack	D
Saturday	C	Any snack	F	Any snack	A
Sunday	B	Any snack	E	Any snack	G

Now let's take a look at how this works in practice. This meal plan is one I made with two of my clients, a married couple, who both work long hours and need quick meals that can keep them full of energy and feeling good.

THE PLAN

Recipe A: Spinach-and-Mushroom-Stuffed Flank Steak (page 203)

Recipe B: Roasted Chickpea Quinoa Buddha Bowl (page 166)

Recipe C: Baked Carrot Cake Oatmeal (page 93)

Recipe D: Crunchy Broccoli Apple Chicken Salad (page 143)

Recipe E: Ham-Loaded Yam (page 176)

Recipe F: Steak Breakfast Fajitas (page 109)

Recipe G: Mole Cabbage Enchiladas with Sweet Potatoes and Black Beans (page 227)

Snacks: Oranges, pears, kiwis, almonds, pumpkin seeds, hard-boiled eggs, Baked Buffalo Wings (page 253), Spicy Salmon Jerky (page 248), and Chocolate-Orange Power Balls (page 250)

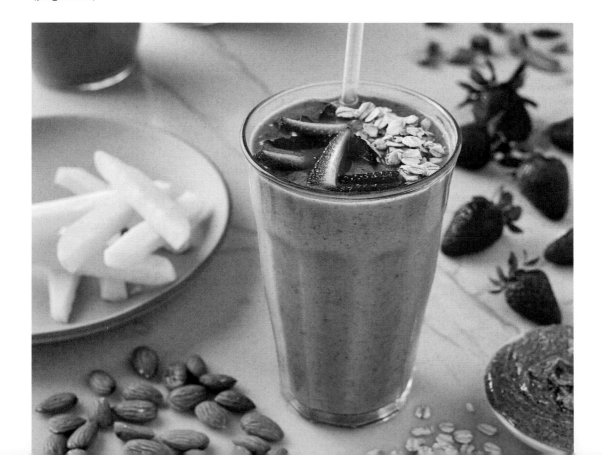

These recipes would spread out over the course of a week like this:

	Breakfast	Snack	Lunch	Snack	Dinner
Monday	C: Baked Carrot Cake Oatmeal	Orange	D: Crunchy Broccoli Apple Chicken Salad	Baked Buffalo Wings	A: Spinach-and-Mushroom-Stuffed Flank Steak
Tuesday	E: Ham-Loaded Yam	Hard-boiled egg	G: Mole Cabbage Enchiladas with Sweet Potatoes and Black Beans	Pear	B: Roasted Chickpea Quinoa Buddha Bowl
Wednesday	C: Baked Carrot Cake Oatmeal	Spicy Salmon Jerky	F: Steak Breakfast Fajitas	Chocolate-Orange Power Balls	D: Crunchy Broccoli Apple Chicken Salad
Thursday	F: Steak Breakfast Fajitas	Orange	B: Roasted Chickpea Quinoa Buddha Bowl	Hard-boiled egg	A: Spinach-and-Mushroom-Stuffed Flank Steak
Friday	E: Ham-Loaded Yam	Almonds	G: Mole Cabbage Enchiladas with Sweet Potatoes and Black Beans	Baked Buffalo Wings	D: Crunchy Broccoli Apple Chicken Salad
Saturday	C: Baked Carrot Cake Oatmeal	Chocolate-Orange Power Balls	F: Steak Breakfast Fajitas	2 kiwis	A: Spinach-and-Mushroom-Stuffed Flank Steak
Sunday	B: Roasted Chickpea Quinoa Buddha Bowl	Spicy Salmon Jerky	E: Ham-Loaded Yam	Apple	G: Mole Cabbage Enchiladas with Sweet Potatoes and Black Beans

To prepare, my clients spent one weekend making twelve servings of each of these recipes. Then they packed them up and labeled them with the recipe name and letter and put them in the freezer. They followed this meal map for two weeks.

It might sound daunting to do all this cooking at once, but you can certainly adjust this for your own needs and schedule. You could do it over two days, maybe making six meals one day and six the next day. Or you could make all the breakfasts at one time on a Saturday or Sunday morning, then all the lunches around noon, then all the dinners in the afternoon. Another way to do this would be to make twelve servings of each recipe whenever it comes up on the schedule for the first time. For example, on Monday morning, my clients could have made twelve servings of Baked Carrot Cake Oatmeal, but packed ten away in the freezer. At lunch that day, they could make twelve servings of Crunchy Broccoli Apple Chicken Salad, packing and freezing ten servings, and so on.

Let's look at another one for good measure. This meal map was for a client who's a busy single woman and rarely gets home before 9 p.m. She needs food she can take with her to the office in addition to quick meals she can make when she gets home after a long day. Here's what we came up with for her:

Recipe A: Vegetarian Baked Lasagna (page 241)

Recipe B: Lentil Veggie Power Bowl (page 170)

Recipe C: Sweet Potato–Pulled Pork Hash (page 117)

Recipe D: Beef Lo Mein (page 209)

Recipe E: Poblano Pork Chili Verde in the Skillet (page 215)

Recipe F: Cashew Soup (page 136)

Recipe G: Spicy Lamb Tagine (page 211)

Snacks: Tangerines, frozen mango, blackberries, hard-boiled eggs, Chocolate-Orange Power Balls (page 250), Cinnamon Chickpeas (page 247), and Grilled Mushroom Skewers with Balsamic Glaze (page 245)

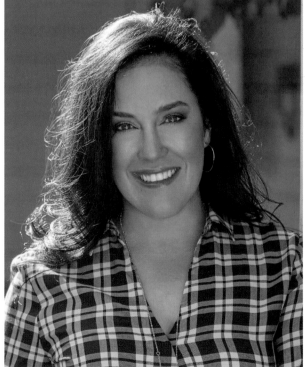

Here's how her meal map looked. She was able to make twelve portions of each recipe, pack and store them, and live off those delicious pre-prepped meals for an entire month—no daily cooking.

	Breakfast	Snack	Lunch	Snack	Dinner
Monday	C: Sweet Potato–Pulled Pork Hash	Tangerines	D: Beef Lo Mein	Hard-boiled egg	A: Vegetarian Baked Lasagna
Tuesday	E: Poblano Pork Chili Verde in the Skillet	Grilled Mushroom Skewers with Balsamic Glaze	G: Spicy Lamb Tagine	Blackberries	B: Lentil Veggie Power Bowl
Wednesday	C: Sweet Potato–Pulled Pork I lash	Chocolate-Orange Power Balls	F: Cashew Soup	Frozen mango	D: Beef Lo Mein
Thursday	F: Cashew Soup	Tangerines	B: Roasted Chickpea Quinoa Buddha Bowl	Grilled Mushroom Skewers with Balsamic Glaze	A: Vegetarian Baked Lasagna
Friday	E: Poblano Pork Chili Verde in the Skillet	Chocolate-Orange Power Balls	G: Spicy Lamb Tagine	Hard-boiled egg	D: Beef Lo Mein
Saturday	C: Sweet Potato–Pulled Pork Hash	Blackberries	F: Cashew Soup	Cinnamon Chickpeas	A: Vegetarian Baked Lasagna
Sunday	B: Lentil Veggie Power Bowl	Grilled Mushroom Skewers with Balsamic Glaze	E: Poblano Pork Chili Verde in the Skillet	Hard-boiled egg	G: Spicy Lamb Tagine

Now It's Your Turn

Just choose any recipe from this book that works with the criteria here:

Recipe A: Dinner recipe: _____

Recipe B: Versatile recipe you might have for breakfast, lunch, or dinner: _____

Recipe C: Breakfast recipe: _____

Recipe D: Recipe that could be lunch or dinner: _____

Recipe E: Recipe that could be breakfast or lunch: _____

Recipe F: Recipe that could be breakfast or lunch: _____

Recipe G: Recipe that could be lunch or dinner: _____

Snacks: _____

Now plug your recipes into this meal map to see how it looks.

	Breakfast	**Snack**	**Lunch**	**Snack**	**Dinner**
Monday	C:		D:		A:
Tuesday	E:		G:		B:
Wednesday	C:		F:		D:
Thursday	F:		B:		A:
Friday	E:		G:		D:
Saturday	C:		F:		A:
Sunday	B:		E:		G:

Now all you have to do is make twelve portions of each recipe, pack them up, label them, and store them in the freezer, and you're ready to go two to four weeks without cooking!

How to Adapt the Recipes
If You Are on One of My Programs

Many of you coming to this book may already be on one of my programs—the Fast Metabolism Diet, one of the Burn plans, one of the programs in *Fast Metabolism Food Rx* or *Metabolism Revolution*, or one of my various cleanses or challenges. If this is you, I want to assure you that you can use many, if not all, of the recipes in this book to further expand your options while on these programs.

If you aren't on one of my other programs but you're considering one, this section will provide a sneak preview into how you might use this cookbook along with those plans. Don't be intimidated. It may sound complex, but once you learn about these programs, it will make much more sense. This guide is really for those who are working through a program and want more options.

Adapting the recipes in this book to your program isn't complicated. It just takes a few extra minutes of planning. Let's start with some basic recipe adaptation rules that apply across the board.

Easy Substitutions

In many of my programs, there are phases or parts where you are more limited in what foods you choose, such as days when you limit fat and focus on carbs or limit carbs and focus on protein. Here are some basic rules that apply to many of the recipes that you may need to adapt:

- **CHOOSE YOUR RECIPE WISELY.** When adapting a recipe, look at the protein and grain requirements on your particular program, part, or phase. This will help you choose a recipe that will be the easiest to adapt. For example, if you're on a phase with only sea-food or vegetable protein options (as on the I-Burn), find seafood or vegetable-based recipes rather than trying to adapt a recipe that depends on steak. If you're on a phase where beef and chicken are allowed but not grains, gravitate more toward the meaty recipes as well as soups and salads where grain is less likely to be featured, rather than trying to adapt a rice dish or oatmeal. If you're on a carb-heavy phase with low fat, look for vegetarian and grain-based recipes rather than a recipe that depends on avocados or olive oil or coconut.

- **YOU CAN STILL USE A RECIPE THAT CONTAINS OIL OR FAT-RICH FOODS** even if your program prohibits the use of oil or fatty food for certain parts of the week by using the following tips:

  - "Sauté" in water or broth instead of oil (stir frequently and add more liquid as it cooks off—this really works and is technically more like braising than sautéing).
  - Substitute ¼ cup unsweetened applesauce or pureed pumpkin for each egg or in equivalent measurements for any oil in any baked recipe.
  - Use parchment paper on your baking sheets, baking pans, loaf pans, or muffin tins instead of greasing them.
  - Replace one whole egg with two egg whites.

- **YOU CAN USE A RECIPE THAT CONTAINS GRAINS OR STARCHES** even if your program prohibits the use of grains or starchy foods for certain parts of the week by making the following modifications:

  - Use spaghetti squash, spiralized zucchini or broccoli stems, or shredded cabbage to replace pasta.
  - Use cauliflower or broccoli "rice" (chopped to resemble rice) to replace rice, quinoa, or any other grain.
  - Use slices of cooked sweet potato or jicama or hollowed-out mushroom caps or cucumbers in place of bread or buns.
  - Leave the grain out of a recipe and increase the vegetables.

It's usually a good idea to reserve truly grain-based dishes like bread or oatmeal for those days when you can have grains.

A PLAN FOR EVERY SITUATION AND LIFESTYLE

One of the things I love about my community is how sophisticated they've become in their knowledge about the metabolism and what works for them. One of my clients is a great example. She likes to hop through my different plans, but whenever she has a question, she asks. Here's what she wrote to our team recently:

> One of the things I like about Haylie's Fast Metabolism community is how much support I get whenever I have a question. Right now, I'm doing her 5-day Fast Metabolism Cleanse. After that, I plan to do a 2-week bootcamp, then the 10-day Fast Metabolism Cleanse, which I've had great success with in the past. But after that, I'm trying to decide what's next. I'm interested in Haylie's Intensives, so I did a quiz on the website to find out which intensive was right for me. My answer was the Phase 1 Intensive, but when I've done the Fast Metabolism Diet in the past, what I really enjoyed was Phase 2. I just breezed through those Phase 2 days, and when I did a Phase 2 Intensive after the last holiday season, I did great with it. What I wanted to know from Haylie's team was: If my quiz results say Phase 1, can I do the Phase 2 Intensive instead because I prefer it? My only concern is that Phase 2 is very low-carb, and from all I've learned in Haylie's books, I don't want to become carb-resistant. Her team was there to help. They advised me that I could do the Phase 2 Intensive, but that it would be good to alternate it with a Phase 1 day before and after. It was the perfect solution. I'm a planner, so I'm really happy to know what's coming and how I'll be eating for the next month. "

Building the Master Metabolism Food List to Match Your Program

Now let's look back at the food list. Each of my programs has its own food list, containing only those foods that are specifically and strategically useful for the goal of that particular program, phase, part, or cleanse. The Master Metabolism Food List in this book (see page 58) is broader, containing all the best metabolism-boosting foods, and this is the list from which the recipes in this book were created. To adapt the recipes, the first thing you will want to do is figure out which food list items you can and can't have to stay compliant with your current program. Here is how I recommend you adapt the Master Metabolism Food List and then the recipes:

1. Make a copy of the Master Metabolism Food List, and put it next to the food list for your current program.

2. Circle all the foods on the Master Metabolism Food List that are also on your program's food list. If your plan has more than one phase (such as the Fast Metabolism Diet Phases 1, 2, and 3), mark the items for each phase. For instance, if you are on FMD, you would mark oatmeal (and other grains) for Phases 1 and 3, but not for Phase 2. You would mark avocado and olive oil for Phase 3, but not for Phases 1 and 2. You would mark leafy greens for Phases 1, 2, and 3.

3. Go to the recipe in this book that you want to make. For any ingredients that are not circled on the list you just made, choose another ingredient in the same category that is circled. For example, if you are on a 10-day cleanse and you want to make the Minty Melon Salad (page 101), you will see that melons aren't on the cleanse list. Instead, you could substitute orchard fruits like peaches, pears, or plums, or make a berry salad with blackberries, blueberries, and cherries.

4. If the recipe contains a food whose entire category is not compliant for your current plan, such as recipes with fat when you are on FMD Phase 1 or fruit on Phase 2, see if you can leave it out. If you can't have oil, you can sauté onions and garlic in vegetable

broth, even though that is not in the same category. Or, you could add applesauce or pumpkin puree in place of fat in a baked recipe.

5. If a recipe is really based on that noncompliant item, like a fruit salad when you are on FMD Phase 2, save that recipe for when you are in a fruit-friendly phase (such as FMD Phase 1).

6. If your program specifies that you eat or drink something particular at each meal (such as on the Burn plans, where you have a specific soup and tea with every meal), just include those as side dishes for the recipe you're making.

Now that you have some basic guidelines, let's look at some of my specific programs and dig in to how this recipe adaptation works.

Example One: The Fast Metabolism Diet (FMD)

If you're on the Fast Metabolism Diet, you know that you do Phase 1 on Monday and Tuesday, Phase 2 on Wednesday and Thursday, and Phase 3 on Friday, Saturday, and Sunday. Here's how you could use the recipes in this cookbook for each phase:

PHASE 1: Let's say you want to make Lemon-Cranberry Bread (page 95) for breakfast while you're on FMD Phase 1. Let's take a look at the ingredients list:

- Instead of using coconut oil to grease the pan, line it with parchment paper.
- Instead of 3 large eggs, use ¾ cup unsweetened applesauce.
- Instead of almond milk, use unsweetened rice milk.
- Instead of olive oil, add additional applesauce or pumpkin puree.
- Instead of cranberries, use blueberries or raspberries.
- Otherwise, follow the instructions as written.

PHASE 2: On this phase, you limit both carbs and fats, focusing on low-fat protein and lots of green vegetables. While you're on Phase 2, you might like the sound of Chicken Pho (page 138) for lunch. Good choice! The only change you would have to make would be to replace the zucchini with spiralized broccoli stalks or cucumbers (peeled and seeded), or maybe green beans or thinly sliced green bell peppers.

But maybe you're more interested in the recipe for Asian Sesame Slaw with Grilled Steak Strips (page 140). Still doable! All you have to do is:

- Eliminate the sesame oil.
- Replace the rice vinegar with apple cider vinegar or white vinegar.
- Replace the Chinese five-spice powder with cinnamon, nutmeg, red pepper flakes, and cloves (or just eliminate it).
- Sauté the steak in water or vegetable broth instead of olive oil.
- Replace the quinoa with more cabbage.
- Replace the snow peas with sliced celery or cucumbers.
- Eliminate the avocado, radishes, scallions, and sesame seeds for the garnish and instead add sliced green chiles or jalapeño slices, shredded lettuce or watercress, and sliced mushrooms, raw or cooked in some water or vegetable broth.
- To add flavor, you could always sprinkle on more coconut aminos.

PHASE 3: This is the easiest of the phases to adapt because it has the longest food list and allows for healthy fats as well as some carbs and protein. But what if you want to make something like Spaghetti Bolognese (page 210) on Phase 3, which doesn't allow for pasta? Just replace those spaghetti noodles with spiralized zucchini or any other squash.

Example Two: The Burn

Now let's say you are doing one of the Burn plans. These are targeted plans to help you break through weight loss plateaus due to inflammation, digestive issues, or hormonal issues. For each plan, you'll have designated teas and soups according to a schedule, but what about when you're having lunch or dinner?

I-BURN: On this plan, the only proteins allowed come from seafood or vegetables, so it would be easiest to choose a vegetarian or seafood recipe. Let's say you want to have the Brazilian Fish Stew (page 230) for dinner. No problem! All you have to do is:

- Instead of salmon, make all the fish haddock or cod.
- Instead of coriander, use fresh cilantro.
- Instead of allspice, use cinnamon or nutmeg.
- Instead of yellow onions, use red onions.
- Use all red bell pepper.
- Instead of coconut cream, use coconut milk.

D-BURN: To manage your digestive issues, you might be on the D-Burn. Maybe you think the Spinach-and-Mushroom-Stuffed Flank Steak (page 203) looks good for dinner. Can do! Just make these changes based on the D-Burn food list:

- Instead of white mushrooms, use shiitakes.
- Instead of rosemary, use oregano.
- Instead of liquid aminos and salt, use beef broth and extra garlic.
- Instead of sprouted-grain bread, use wild rice or quinoa.
- Instead of Brussels sprouts, use bok choy.

H-BURN: When your hormones are giving you trouble, the H-Burn can come to the rescue, and so can this cookbook. This plan avoids nightshade vegetables, so look for recipes that don't depend on peppers or tomatoes—although you can always swap them out for cabbage, asparagus, spinach, zucchini, and mushrooms. Maybe you're eyeing the Slow Cooker Roasted Mediterranean Chicken (page 188). Just make these substitutions based on your food list:

- Instead of the red and green bell peppers, use 1 cup each of green beans and chopped kale.
- Instead of the cherry tomatoes, increase the zucchini by 1 cup or add 1 cup chopped yellow squash.
- Instead of the cannellini beans, add an additional cup of mushrooms or an additional chicken breast.

Example Three: Metabolism Revolution (MR)

If you're doing Metabolism Revolution, you have the same food list for all meal maps and parts. It's about when you eat what. To comply with this plan, look at your meal map and see how many servings of what categories you need.

For example, let's say you have been assigned to Meal Map B. In the first half of the week, your dinner will consist of:

1 serving protein
2 servings vegetables
1 serving non-grain-based complex carbs

First, you know your carb serving can't be a grain, so look for a recipe that doesn't rely on grain. What about White Chicken Chili (page 191)? Let's try it:

- The chicken takes care of your protein serving.
- Double up the vegetables to get your two servings.
- The beans are your non-grain-based carbs.

Easy! Now, what about the second half of the week? Let's look at Meal Map C this time. Your requirements for dinner are:

1 serving protein
2 servings vegetables
2 servings healthy fat

Now you want to look for a low-carb recipe that focuses on protein but doesn't need to limit fat. Let's see what we can do with the Slow Cooker Greek Drumsticks with Asparagus (page 195):

- The chicken takes care of the protein.
- Double the asparagus or add a side salad to get your two vegetable servings.
- For your fat, you could make either Cashew Sour Cream (page 263) or Coconut Sour Cream (page 263).

Example Four: The 10-Day Fast Metabolism Cleanse

Let's do one more. Maybe you're on my Fast Metabolism Cleanse, using the cleanse shake along with designated meals. You don't have to be limited to the meals in the cleanse plan as long as you stick to the cleanse food list. There are plenty of options on the cleanse food list. Here's how you might do Day 3 on the cleanse, when you have three shakes, one meal, and one snack:

Breakfast: Cleanse shake
Snack: Blueberries and carrots
Lunch: Cleanse shake
Snack: Cleanse shake
Dinner: The cleanse recommends recipes, but you might be ready for a change. How about Chicken and Black Bean Tortilla Soup (page 192)? It doesn't even need any changes. How about the Taco Pasta Casserole (page 207)? Sure, why not? All you have to do is:

- Replace the ground beef with ground buffalo.
- Replace the brown rice penne with brown rice (you can call it "Taco Rice Casserole"), spaghetti squash, or spiralized zucchini.

As you can see, adapting the recipes in this cookbook for your program is really pretty straightforward. It's all about the food lists and, in some cases, the preparation techniques. Not every single recipe will work for every single phase, part, or plan, but the recipes in this cookbook will give you many more options to make whatever program you are on more fun, interesting, and even more sustainable. Now . . . let's get cooking!

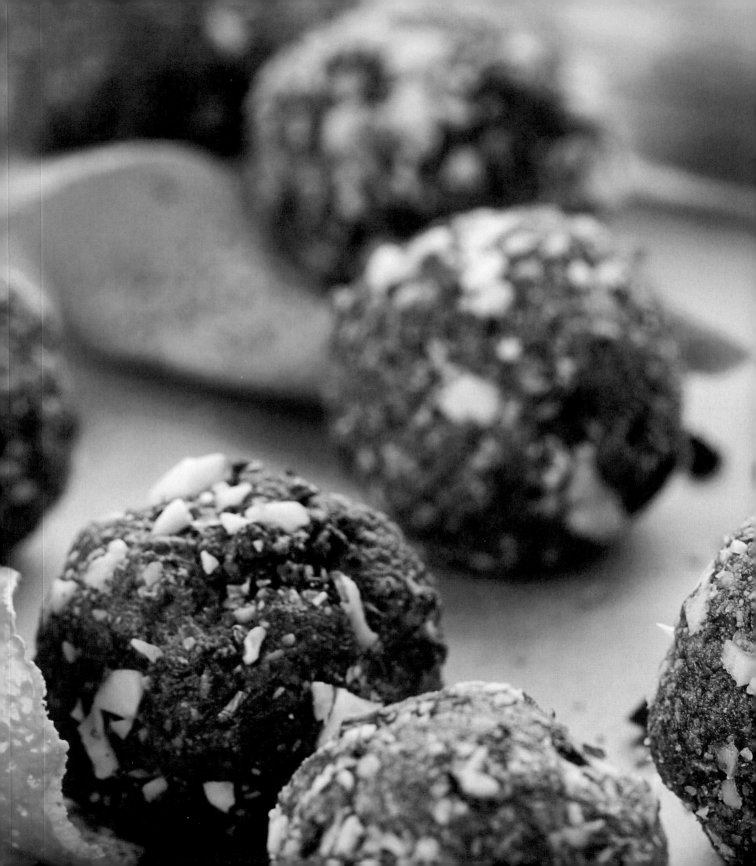

PART II

RECIPES FOR A FAST METABOLISM

BREAKFASTS

Spa Smoothie

Serves 1

IN a high-powered blender, combine all the ingredients and blend until smooth, adding a little more water if it's too thick.

2 handfuls ice

1 cup water, plus more if needed

1 cup sliced cucumber

½ cup fresh spinach

¼ cup fresh mint

¼ cup coarsely chopped fresh basil

2 egg whites, from hard-boiled eggs, or ¼ cup cooked 100% liquid egg whites

1 lemon, peeled and seeded

1 (1-inch) piece fresh ginger, peeled and coarsely chopped

Stevia or xylitol (optional)

Strawberry Rhubarb Pie Smoothie

Serves 1

IN a high-powered blender, combine all the ingredients and blend until smooth, adding a little water if it's too thick.

1 cup frozen strawberries

¾ cup unsweetened vanilla almond milk

½ cup frozen rhubarb

⅛ cup old-fashioned oats

1 tablespoon raw almond butter or cashews

Stevia or xylitol (optional)

1½ cups chopped peeled jicama

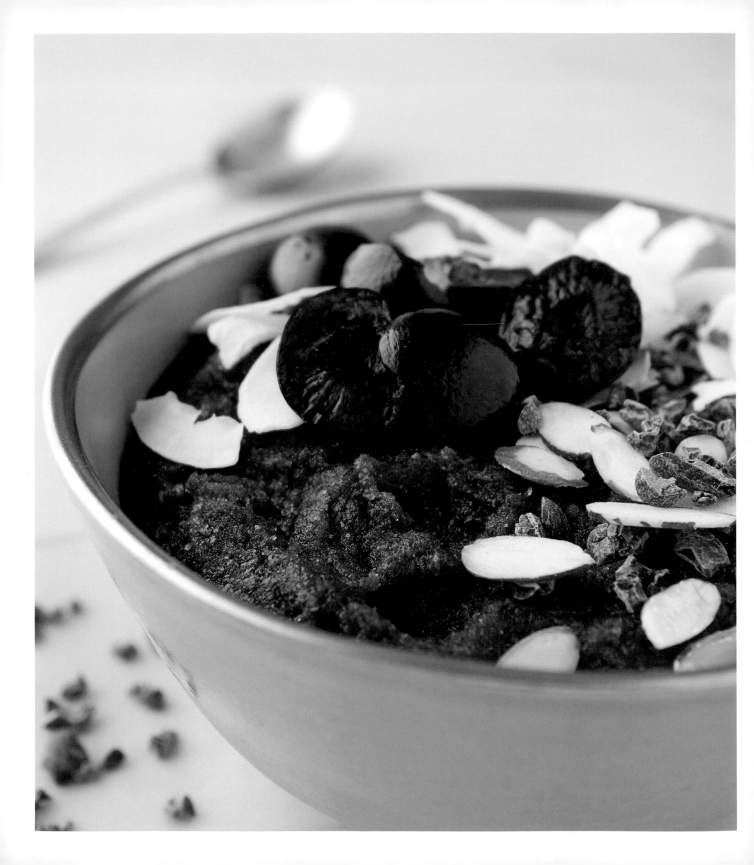

Cherry Almond Smoothie Bowl

Serves 2

IN a high-powered blender, combine the cherries, cauliflower, and coconut water and blend until smooth, adding a little water if it's too thick. Pour the smoothie mixture into two bowls and evenly divide the toppings between them.

VARIATIONS
- Make this smoothie bowl with different combinations of fruits and nuts, such as peaches and pecans, plums and hazelnuts, or mangoes and macadamias.

2 cups frozen pitted cherries

1 cup frozen cauliflower florets

¾ cup unsweetened coconut water

Topping

8 whole pitted cherries, fresh or thawed frozen

¼ cup unsweetened coconut flakes

¼ cup sliced almonds

¼ cup raw cacao nibs

Crispy Quinoa Chia Bars

Serves 6

6 ripe apricots, pitted

1 tablespoon water

½ cup nut or seed butter

2 cups puffed quinoa

¼ cup coconut oil, melted

2 tablespoons chia seeds

½ teaspoon pure vanilla extract

¼ teaspoon sea salt

LINE an 8- or 9-inch square baking pan with parchment paper.

IN a high-powered blender, puree the apricots and water. Add the nut or seed butter. Blend until pureed.

IN a large bowl, combine the puffed quinoa, apricot mixture, melted coconut oil, chia seeds, vanilla, and salt. Stir until everything is evenly mixed. Put the quinoa mixture into the prepared pan and spread it evenly to the edges, pressing it down with your fingers.

PUT the pan in the refrigerator for at least 40 minutes, or until firm. Meanwhile, cut 6 strips of parchment paper, about 4×6 inches each.

CUT the chilled mixture into 6 rectangles. Put each bar on a strip of parchment and wrap the long ends around the bar. Serve immediately or store in an airtight container in the refrigerator for up to 3 days.

VARIATION
- Use puffed brown rice instead of quinoa.

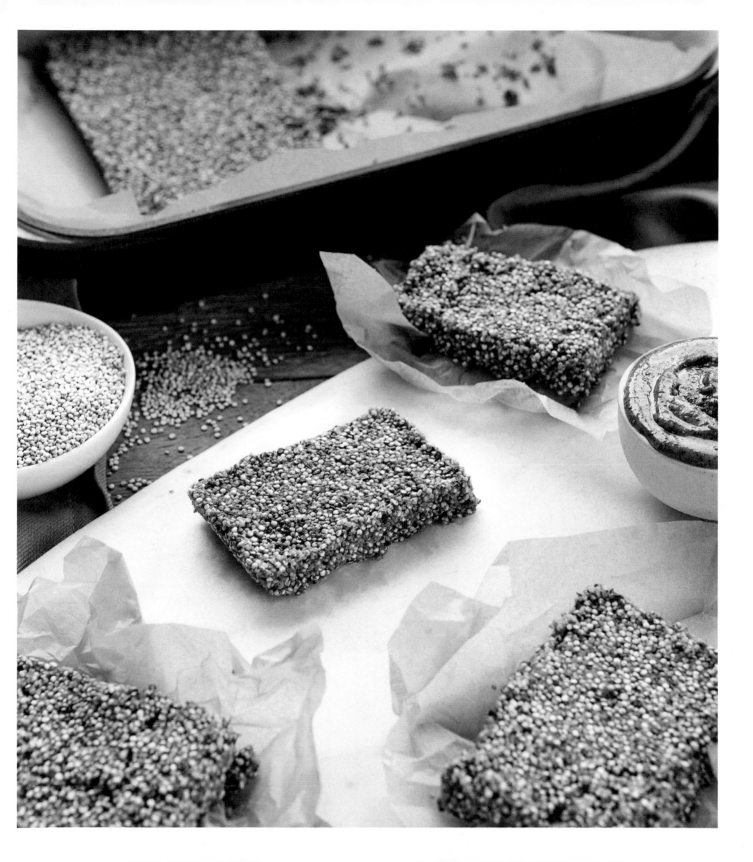

Mint Chocolate Chip Smoothie Bowl

Serves 1

IN a blender, combine the cauliflower, spinach, almond milk, cashews, mint oil (if using), and stevia or xylitol (if using). Blend for 2 minutes, adding a little water if it's too thick. Add half the cacao nibs and pulse a few times. Pour the mixture into a bowl. Top with the remaining cacao nibs, the mint leaves (if using), and coconut flakes.

1 cup fresh or frozen cauliflower florets (use frozen for a frostier bowl)

1 cup fresh or frozen baby spinach (use frozen for a frostier bowl)

1 cup unsweetened almond milk

2 tablespoons raw cashews

¼ cup chopped fresh mint leaves, or 4 drops food-grade peppermint essential oil

Stevia or xylitol (optional)

2 tablespoons raw cacao nibs

Unsweetened coconut flakes, for garnish

Blackberry Crumble Breakfast Bars

Serves 8

IN a medium saucepan, combine the blackberries, xylitol (if using), lemon zest, and lemon juice. Cook over medium-high heat, stirring and pressing on the berries to break them up. Simmer until slightly thickened, about 3 minutes, then reduce the heat to low. Cook for 3 minutes more, then remove the pan from the heat and stir in the chia seeds. Set aside to cool.

PREHEAT the oven to 350°F. Line an 8-inch square baking pan with parchment paper. Grease the parchment with 1 teaspoon of the coconut oil.

MAKE THE CRUST: In a food processor, combine the oat flour, nuts, 2 tablespoons coconut oil, water, vanilla, and salt. Pulse until the mixture looks crumbly. Transfer it to the prepared pan and press it into an even layer. Bake for 12 minutes, or until the crust just begins to brown. Remove from the oven, but the leave the oven on.

MAKE THE TOPPING: Without cleaning the food processor, combine the nuts, coconut, oats, xylitol, coconut oil, cinnamon, and salt in the bowl. Pulse until the mixture looks crumbly.

DROP spoonfuls of the blackberry filling evenly over the crust, then spread it carefully. Sprinkle the topping over the filling. Bake for 15 minutes, or until golden brown. Remove from the oven and let cool. When the bars are completely cool, cut them into 8 squares. Store in an airtight container in the refrigerator for up to 3 days.

VARIATIONS

- Substitute any other berries, or chopped apples, peaches, or plums.

Filling

2 cups frozen blackberries

2 tablespoons xylitol (optional)

Pinch of lemon zest

1 tablespoon fresh lemon juice

1 tablespoon chia seeds

Crust

2 tablespoons plus 1 teaspoon coconut oil

1 cup oat flour

¼ cup raw walnuts or almonds

1 tablespoon water

1 teaspoon pure vanilla extract

¼ teaspoon sea salt

Topping

¾ cup raw walnuts or almonds

½ cup unsweetened shredded coconut

¼ cup quick-cooking oats

2 tablespoons xylitol

1 tablespoon coconut oil

½ teaspoon ground cinnamon

¼ teaspoon sea salt

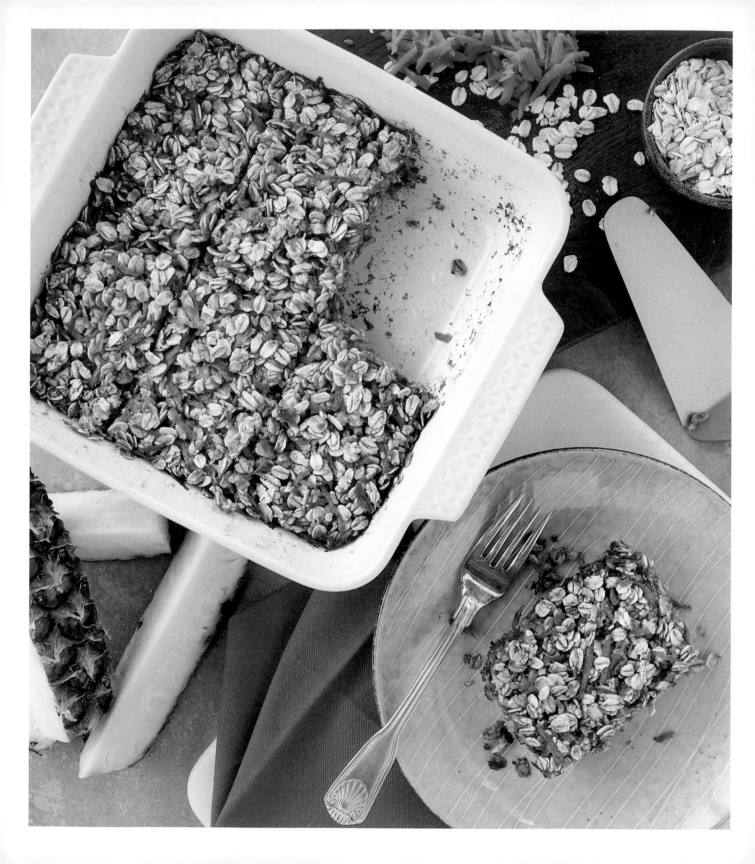

Baked Carrot Cake Oatmeal

Serves 6

PREHEAT the oven to 350°F. Line an 8-inch square baking pan with a piece of parchment paper cut to fit.

IN a large bowl, combine the oats, carrot, pineapple, cinnamon, ginger, baking powder, nutmeg, and salt and stir until well mixed.

IN a medium bowl, whisk together the milk, xylitol, egg, and vanilla until smooth.

POUR the milk mixture into the flour mixture and stir gently until fully combined. Pour the batter into the prepared pan and spread it to cover the bottom evenly.

BAKE for about 40 minutes, or until golden brown and set in the middle. Remove from the oven and cool for 5 minutes, then cut into 6 squares and serve.

2½ cups old-fashioned oats

1½ cups grated carrots

½ cup chopped pineapple

2 teaspoons ground cinnamon

1 teaspoon ground ginger

1 teaspoon baking powder

¼ teaspoon ground nutmeg

¼ teaspoon sea salt

1 cup unsweetened oat milk or rice milk

½ cup xylitol, or more to taste

1 large egg

2 teaspoons pure vanilla extract

Chai-Spiced Overnight Oats

Serves 1

COMBINE the oats, almond milk, flaxseed, chia seeds, xylitol, cinnamon, cardamom, ginger, nutmeg, and vanilla in a container with a lid (a Mason jar is a good option) and stir to mix everything evenly. Cover and refrigerate overnight.

IN the morning, stir and top with fruit and nuts.

½ cup old-fashioned oats

½ cup unsweetened almond milk

1½ teaspoons ground flaxseed

1½ teaspoons chia seeds

1½ teaspoons xylitol

⅛ teaspoon ground cinnamon

⅛ teaspoon ground cardamom

⅛ teaspoon ground ginger

⅛ teaspoon ground nutmeg

⅛ teaspoon pure vanilla extract

1 cup FMD-approved fruit (any type)

3 tablespoons nuts (any type)

Lemon-Cranberry Bread

Makes one 8×5-inch loaf

PREHEAT the oven to 350°F. Line an 8×5-inch loaf pan with parchment paper and grease any exposed sides with coconut oil.

IN a large bowl, stir together the almond flour, coconut flour, lemon zest, baking soda, and salt to combine. Add the eggs, xylitol (if using), almond milk, olive oil, and vanilla. Mix well. Gently stir in the cranberries.

LET the batter sit for 5 minutes or so to give the coconut flour time to absorb the liquids. Transfer the batter to the prepared loaf pan and bake for 40 minutes, or until the top is golden brown and a toothpick inserted into the center of the bread comes out clean.

COOL completely, then glaze, if desired.

TO make the glaze, whiz the xylitol in a blender until it is broken down to a fine powder. Put the xylitol in a small bowl. Stir in the lemon juice, and drizzle the glaze over the bread.

Coconut oil, for greasing the pan

¾ cup almond flour

¼ cup coconut flour

1 tablespoon lemon zest

½ teaspoon baking soda

¼ teaspoon sea salt

3 large eggs

⅓ cup xylitol (optional)

¼ cup unsweetened almond milk

2 tablespoons olive oil

2 teaspoons pure vanilla extract

1 cup fresh cranberries, coarsely chopped

Glaze (optional)

½ cup xylitol

1 tablespoon fresh lemon juice

Raspberry Cacao Slow Cooker Bread Pudding

Serves 8

IN a medium bowl, whisk together the milk, eggs, xylitol, and vanilla.

PUT the bread cubes and raspberries in a slow cooker, then toss gently together. Sprinkle the cacao nibs evenly over the top. Pour the milk mixture evenly over the top. Cover and cook on high for 2 hours, or until the bread pudding turns golden brown. Scoop out into bowls and serve each bowl topped with a dollop of coconut whipped cream, a few fresh raspberries, and a sprinkle of cinnamon.

VARIATIONS

- This is also good with strawberries, blackberries, or a mixed berry combo.

1½ cups unsweetened oat milk or rice milk

4 large eggs

2 tablespoons xylitol or lo han (monk fruit)

2 teaspoons pure vanilla extract

10 slices sprouted-grain bread, cut into cubes

2 cups fresh raspberries

½ cup raw cacao nibs

Coconut Whipped Cream (page 266), for serving

Fresh raspberries, for serving

Ground cinnamon, for garnish

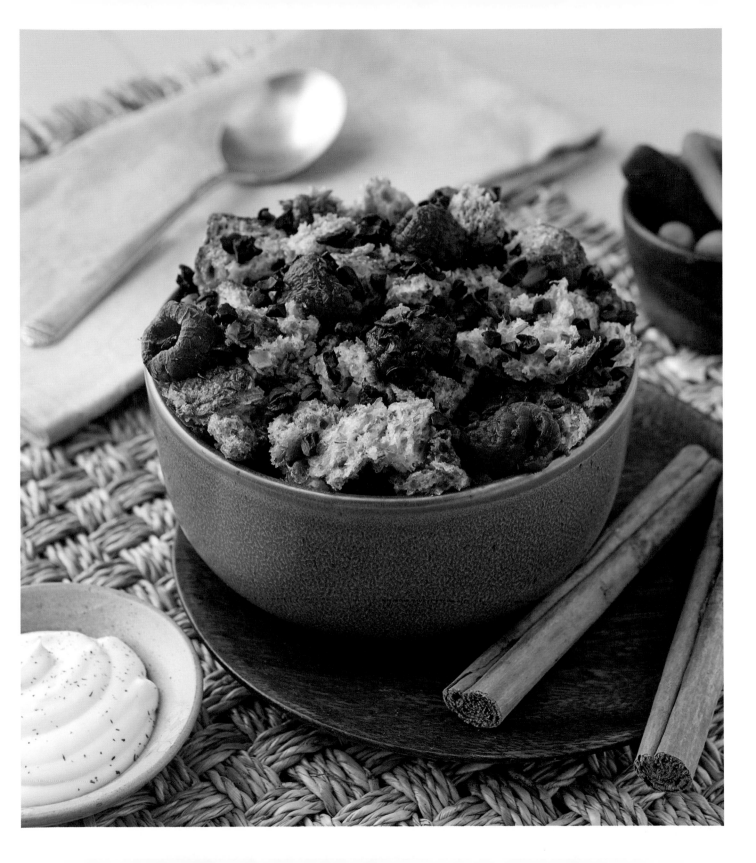

Stuffed Sweet Potato,
Four Ways

Serves 1

---

1 sweet potato, baked

Avocado Version
Top your sweet potato with:

¼ avocado, cut into small cubes

2 tablespoons finely chopped red onion

1 small tomato, chopped

Almond Butter Version
Top your sweet potato with:

1 small apple, cored and chopped

1 tablespoon almond butter, heated and mixed
with 1 teaspoon water, drizzled over the apple

Dash of ground cinnamon

1 tablespoon raw pumpkin seeds (pepitas)

Smoked Salmon Version
Top your sweet potato with:

6 ounces smoked salmon, chopped

½ cup peeled, seeded, and chopped cucumber

2 tablespoons finely chopped red onion

1 tablespoon capers

Chicken Sausage Version
Top your sweet potato with:

4 ounces nitrate-free, no-sugar-added cooked
chicken sausage

1 cup chopped kale, sautéed

½ cup diced red bell pepper, sautéed

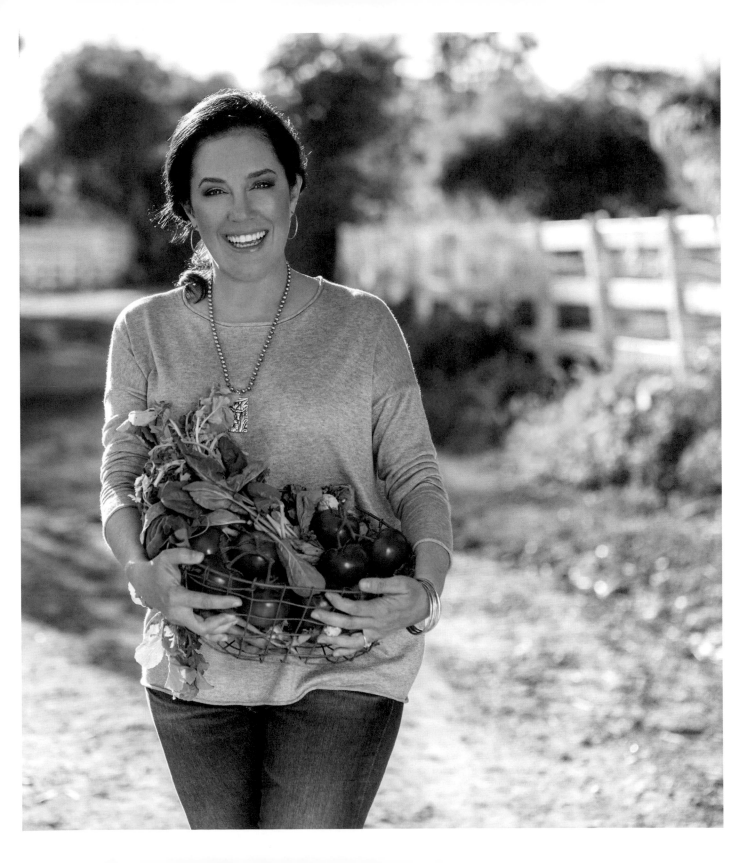

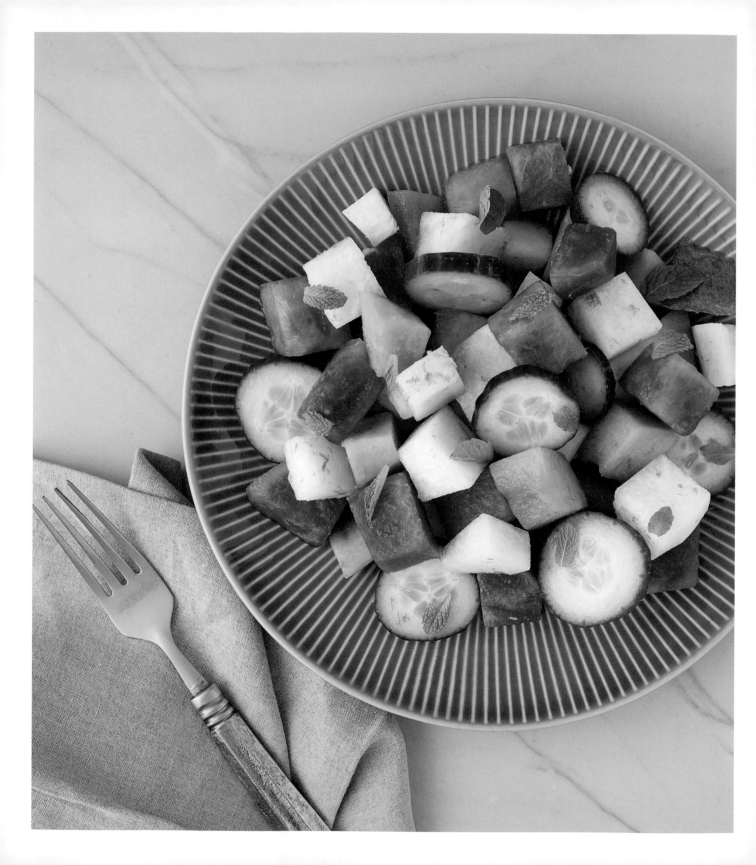

Minty Melon Salad

Serves 6

IN a large serving bowl, combine the watermelon, cantaloupe, honeydew, jicama, and cucumber. In a small bowl, combine the lime zest, lime juice, and stevia (if using), then pour it over the melon mixture and toss to coat. Sprinkle with the mint and salt just before serving.

2 cups watermelon cubes

2 cups cantaloupe cubes

2 cups honeydew melon cubes

2 cups jicama cubes

1 cup sliced cucumber

4 teaspoons lime zest

2 tablespoons fresh lime juice

8 drops liquid stevia (optional)

2 tablespoons finely chopped fresh mint leaves

¼ teaspoon sea salt

VARIATION

- Leave out the stevia and drizzle the salad with 6 tablespoons balsamic vinegar reduction (see below) just before serving

HOW TO MAKE BALSAMIC VINEGAR REDUCTION

Balsamic vinegar is already rich and thick-ish, but it's simple to make it into a rich syrup that is awesome drizzled on salads and fruit. Put twice the amount you need in a small saucepan and let it cook over medium-low heat until it has reduced in volume by half. Or use a large saucepan and reduce 2 cups vinegar down to 1 cup, then store what you don't use in an airtight container in the refrigerator for up to 2 weeks.

Black- and Blueberry Quinoa Breakfast Salad

Serves 4

IN a large bowl, gently toss together the quinoa, blackberries, blueberries, and chia seeds.

IN a small bowl, whisk together the lemon zest, lemon juice, xylitol (if using) and vanilla. Drizzle the mixture over the quinoa and berries. Sprinkle the cinnamon on top of everything and gently mix to distribute the lemon juice mixture and cinnamon. Divide the salad among four bowls and sprinkle 1 tablespoon of the almonds over each bowl.

1 cup cooked tricolor quinoa

1 cup fresh blackberries

1 cup fresh blueberries

¼ cup chia seeds

Zest and juice of 1 lemon

1 tablespoon xylitol (optional)

1 teaspoon pure vanilla extract

½ teaspoon ground cinnamon

4 tablespoons sliced raw almonds

Spicy Fruit Salad

Serves 4

IN a large bowl, combine the mango, papaya, jicama, watermelon, and cucumber cubes. Toss gently to combine, then stir in the orange. Mix until everything is combined. Drizzle the lime juice over the fruit mixture, then sprinkle the cilantro, chili powder, and salt over the top. Toss everything together again to mix well. Chill for at least 30 minutes before serving.

VARIATION

- For a sweeter, more tropical version of this salad, use regular papaya and replace the chili powder with ground cinnamon and/or unsweetened coconut flakes.

1 large mango, peeled, seeded, and cut into small cubes

1 small to medium Mexican papaya, peeled, seeded, and cut into small cubes

1 jicama (about ½ pound), peeled and cut into small cubes

1 cup watermelon cubes

1 medium cucumber, peeled, seeded, and cut into small cubes

½ orange or 1 small clementine, peeled, seeded, sectioned, and coarsely chopped

1 tablespoon fresh lime juice

1 tablespoon finely chopped fresh cilantro

¼ to ½ teaspoon chili powder

Pinch of sea salt, or to taste

Southwest Breakfast Salad with Cilantro-Lime Dressing

Serves 4

BROWN the chicken sausages in a skillet. Slice them.

LAYER the greens, beans, tomatoes, bell pepper, onion, and avocado in four large bowls, dividing them evenly, then top with the sausage.

MAKE the vinaigrette: In a blender, combine the cilantro, olive oil, garlic, tomatillo, lime juice, vinegar, and xylitol and blend until smooth.

DRIZZLE the vinaigrette over the salads, dividing it evenly, and serve.

VARIATIONS

- Use black beans instead of pinto beans.
- Add 1 cup (total for all servings) of cooked brown rice on top of the greens, before the beans.
- Add 1 pound (total for all servings) of any cooked meat or seafood, such as steak strips, chicken strips, or shrimp, on top of the greens, instead of or in addition to the pinto beans.

4 nitrate-free, no-sugar-added cooked chicken sausages

8 cups spring greens

1 (15-ounce) can pinto beans, drained and rinsed

1 cup grape tomatoes, halved

1 green bell pepper, diced

1 medium red onion, diced

1 avocado, sliced

Cilantro-Lime Vinaigrette

1 bunch fresh cilantro

6 tablespoons extra-virgin olive oil

2 garlic cloves, minced

½ fresh tomatillo, husked and well rinsed

Juice of 2 limes

1 tablespoon unseasoned rice vinegar

1½ teaspoons xylitol, or to taste

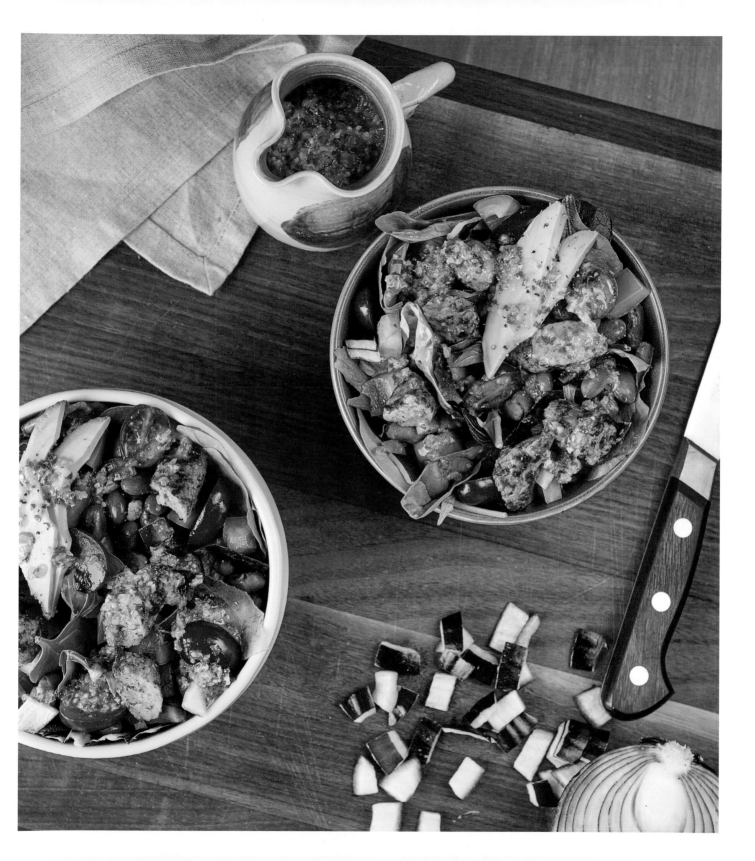

Stone Fruit–Cucumber Salad

Serves 2

IN a jar with a lid, combine the lime juice, olive oil, garlic, cardamom, cumin, salt, and pepper. Put on the lid and shake well to combine.

IN a large bowl, combine the cucumber, peaches, plums, quinoa, parsley, and basil. Drizzle with the dressing and toss until everything is combined. Divide between two bowls and sprinkle the pine nuts on top.

VARIATIONS

- Try brown rice instead of quinoa.
- Add 1 cup diced cooked chicken.
- Instead of stone fruits, you could make this salad with a mix of blueberries, raspberries, and/or blackberries.

¼ cup fresh lime juice

1 tablespoon olive oil

1 garlic clove, minced

½ teaspoon ground cardamom

½ teaspoon ground cumin

¼ teaspoon sea salt

⅛ teaspoon freshly ground black pepper

1 medium English cucumber, cut into small cubes

2 medium peaches or nectarines, pitted and cut into 1-inch pieces

2 red or purple plums, pitted and cut into 1-inch pieces

1 cup cooked tricolor quinoa

¼ cup chopped fresh parsley leaves

¼ cup chopped fresh basil leaves

1 tablespoon raw pine nuts

Crustless Quiche

Serves 6

IN a medium saucepan, melt the coconut oil over medium heat. Add the onion and cook until the onion is soft and translucent, then add the mushrooms. Cover and let the mixture sweat for about 8 minutes, but don't let the onions brown. Stir in the broth and turn the heat to medium-high. Bring to a boil. Immediately reduce the heat to medium-low and simmer, covered, for 1 hour. Let cool, then transfer to a blender and blend until smooth.

PREHEAT the oven to 350°F. Lightly grease a large glass or ceramic pie plate with coconut oil.

PUT the broccoli, scallions, and cheese (if using) in the bottom of the prepared plate.

IN a bowl, beat the eggs, then whisk in the mushroom puree, salt, and pepper. Pour evenly over the cheese.

BAKE for 35 to 45 minutes, until a knife inserted into the center comes out clean.

LET stand for 10 minutes before slicing and serving.

1½ teaspoons coconut oil, plus more for greasing the pan

¼ cup thinly sliced onion

6 ounces white mushrooms, sliced

¾ cup chicken broth or vegetable broth

2 (10-ounce) packages frozen broccoli, chopped, cooked, and well drained

⅓ cup chopped scallions

6 ounces shredded almond cheese or other dairy-free, soy-free cheese (store-bought, or make your own with the recipe on page 264; optional)

6 large eggs

¼ teaspoon sea salt

⅛ teaspoon freshly ground black pepper

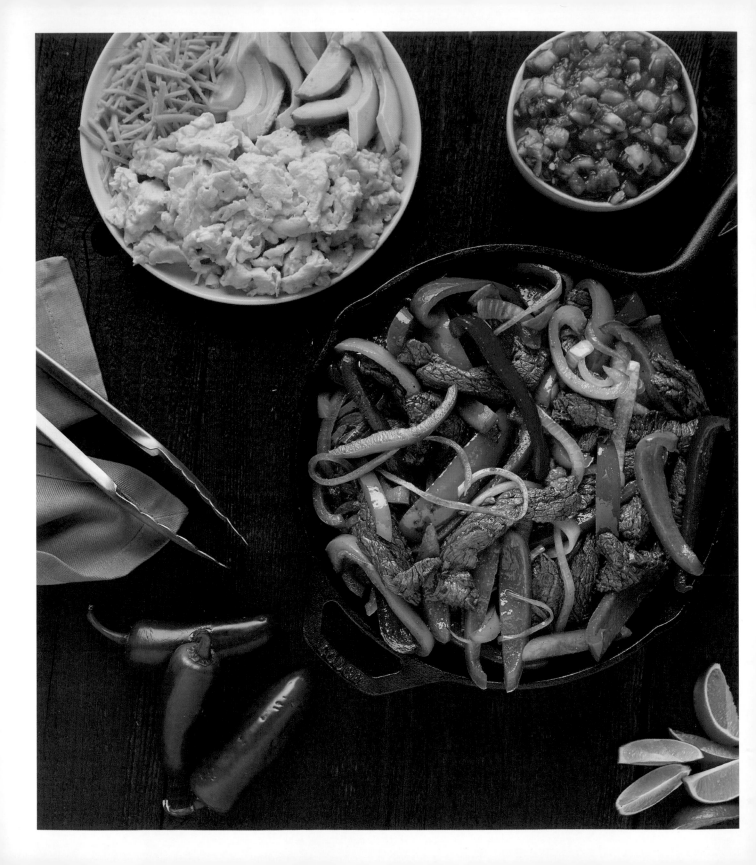

Steak Breakfast Fajitas

Serves 6

PUT the steak in a shallow pan and sprinkle with the vinegar, liquid aminos, chili powder, and black pepper. Set aside to marinate.

IN a large skillet, heat the coconut oil over medium-high heat. When the oil is warm, add the bell peppers and onions. Sauté until the vegetables just begin to soften, about 5 minutes. Add the paprika, garlic powder, cayenne, lime juice, and salt. Stir to combine and cook, stirring occasionally, for 5 minutes more. Remove from the heat and set aside.

DISCARD the marinade and grill or broil the steak for 3 minutes on each side, then remove from the heat. Cover the steak and let it rest for 10 minutes.

MEANWHILE, heat a nonstick skillet over medium heat. Scramble the eggs to your desired level of doneness.

SLICE the steak into strips. Divide the onion-pepper mixture among six plates. Top them evenly with the steak strips, scrambled eggs, avocado slices, salsa, and cheese (if using).

VARIATIONS

- Make chicken or shrimp fajitas, or use a combination of meats.
- Warm sprouted-grain tortillas and serve them on the side, and/or serve with brown rice and black beans on the side.
- For a vegetarian version, leave out the meat and add 2 cups sliced mushrooms.

½ pound skirt or flank steak

½ cup red wine vinegar

¼ cup liquid aminos

1 teaspoon chili powder or chipotle powder

1 teaspoon freshly ground black pepper

1 tablespoon coconut oil

4 cups sliced bell peppers, any color (or a combination)

2 cups white onion slices, broken up into strips

1 tablespoon paprika or smoked paprika

1½ teaspoons garlic powder

1 teaspoon cayenne pepper, or to taste

Juice of ½ lime

1 teaspoon sea salt

4 large eggs

2 avocados, sliced

½ cup salsa

½ cup shredded almond cheese or other dairy-free, soy-free cheese (store-bought, or make your own with the recipe on page 264; optional)

Garden Egg Foo Yung

Serves 6

IN a large bowl, beat the eggs until combined. Add the chicken, bok choy, bean sprouts, bell pepper, squash, broccoli, mushrooms, onion, tamari, garlic powder, and black pepper. Set aside.

PREHEAT the oven to 170°F. Line a baking sheet with parchment paper.

MAKE the sauce: In a small saucepan, whisk together the broth, liquid aminos, rice vinegar, and arrowroot mixture. Cook over medium-high heat, stirring often, until the sauce bubbles, then continue to cook, stirring often, until the sauce thickens, about 3 minutes. Remove from the heat and stir in the sesame oil.

HEAT a small 6-inch nonstick skillet with a lid (or line a regular skillet with parchment paper) over medium heat. Pour in about ⅔ cup of the egg mixture. Cook for about 3 minutes, or until the bottom looks set. Cover the pan and cook for 3 minutes more, or until the top looks set. Transfer the egg pancake to the prepared baking sheet and put it in the oven to keep warm. Repeat to make a total of 12 pancakes.

DIVIDE the spinach among six plates. Put two pancakes on each plate on top of the spinach. Top with the sauce and serve.

8 large eggs

6 ounces boneless, skinless chicken thighs, cooked and shredded

1 cup chopped bok choy

1 cup bean sprouts

1 cup finely chopped orange (or any color) bell pepper

1 cup cubed yellow squash

½ cup chopped broccoli

½ cup chopped mushrooms

½ yellow onion, chopped

1 tablespoon tamari

½ teaspoon garlic powder

¼ teaspoon freshly ground black pepper

Sauce

1 cup chicken broth

2 tablespoons liquid aminos

1 tablespoon plain (unseasoned) rice vinegar

1 tablespoon arrowroot powder, mixed with 1 tablespoon water

1 teaspoon sesame oil

6 cups fresh spinach, for serving

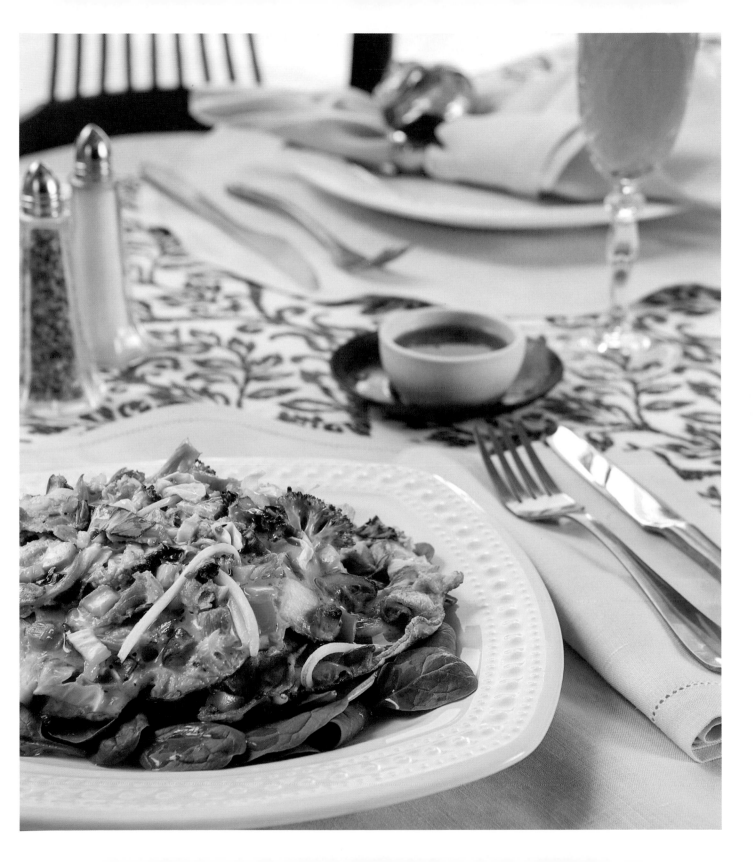

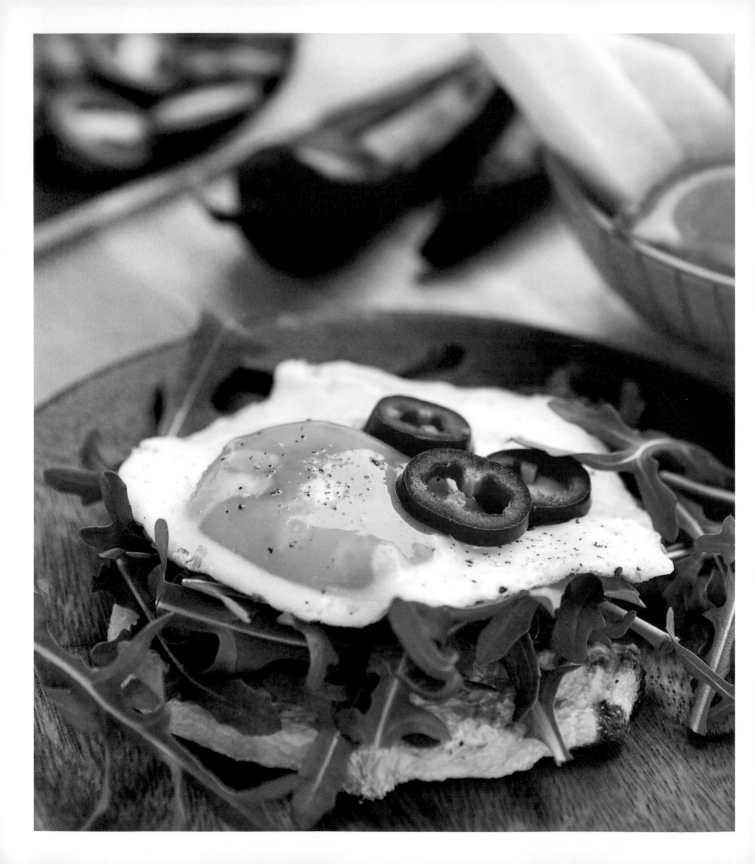

Jicama Toast with Egg

Serves 1

CUT a ¼-inch-thick slice from the center (the widest part) of the jicama. Cut the remaining jicama into sticks and set aside. Put the jicama slice in the toaster on the highest setting. Toast it for two cycles, or until it is lightly browned on both sides.

MEANWHILE, in a nonstick skillet, fry the egg to your liking.

PUT the toasted jicama slice on a plate. Top with the arugula, then the egg, then the jalapeño (if using). Season with salt and pepper, and serve with a lime wedge and the jicama sticks on the side.

1 small jicama, peeled

1 large egg

1 cup arugula or microgreens

1 tablespoon sliced jalapeño (optional)

Sea salt and freshly ground black pepper

1 lime wedge, for garnish

Sweet Potato Chive Waffles with Poached Egg and Savory Salsa "Syrup"

Serves 2

PREHEAT a waffle iron on high.

IN a medium bowl, combine the sweet potato, chives, salt, and pepper and toss to combine. In a small bowl, beat one egg, then add it to the sweet potato mixture, stirring until it is fully incorporated. Coat or spray the waffle iron with the grapeseed oil. Spread half the sweet potato mixture evenly over the waffle iron plate. Close and cook until the waffle iron says it's done.

MEANWHILE, poach the remaining 2 eggs (see "How to Poach an Egg," page 116).

USING a spatula, carefully remove the waffle from the waffle iron and put it on a plate. Repeat with the remaining sweet potato mixture.

TOP each waffle with a poached egg. Drizzle the pureed salsa "syrup" over the eggs. Serve with the tomato slices on the side.

1 large sweet potato, grated and packed in paper towels to absorb moisture (about 2 packed cups)

¼ cup chopped fresh chives

½ teaspoon sea salt

Dash of freshly ground black pepper

3 large eggs

1 teaspoon grapeseed oil

½ cup of your favorite salsa, pureed in a blender

1½ cups tomato slices

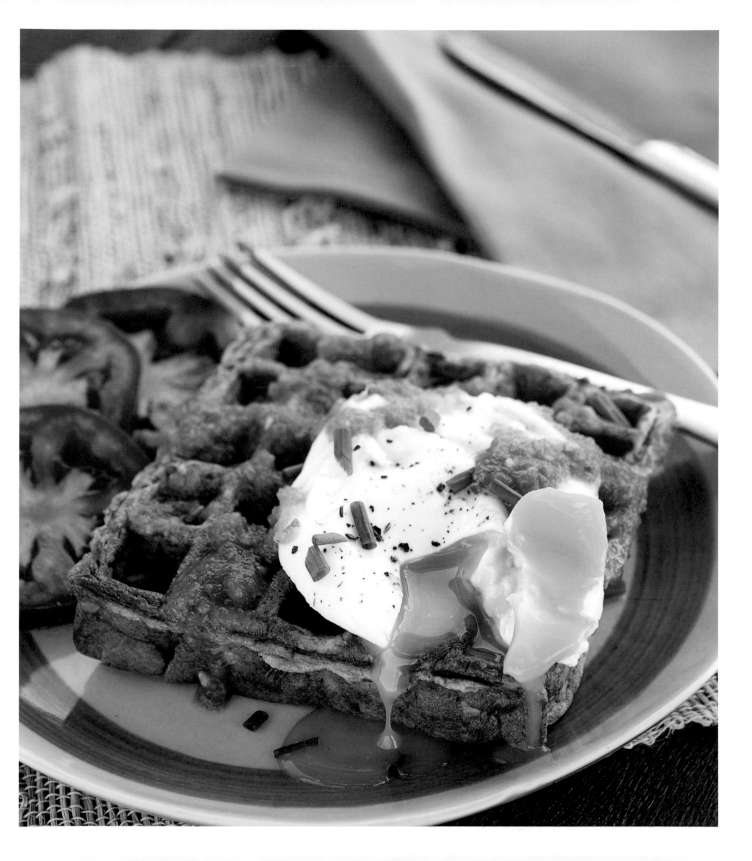

How to Poach an Egg

Of all the ways to cook eggs, poaching seems to be the method most shrouded in mystery. There are many different so-called "secrets" to making the perfect poached egg. Probably the easiest is with an egg poacher—these inexpensive little gadgets make poached eggs quickly, no boiling water necessary. However, if you want to make them the old-fashioned way, the method below works best:

1. Use the freshest eggs you can find.

2. Working with one egg at a time, break the egg into a fine-mesh strainer to get rid of the most liquid parts of the egg white, then tip it carefully into a small bowl or ramekin. (Use a separate bowl or ramekin for each egg you're poaching.)

3. Fill a medium saucepan halfway full with water and bring the water to a boil.

4. When it is boiling, add 2 tablespoons white vinegar. Do not add salt. Reduce the heat to low.

5. Using a spoon, swirl the water around a few times to create a vortex effect, then carefully pour the egg right into the middle of the vortex.

6. Poach the egg for 3 to 4 minutes, depending on how done you like your egg to be.

7. Scoop it out with a slotted spoon and set it on a paper-towel-lined plate.

8. Repeat to cook any additional eggs. Serve warm.

You could cook more than one egg at a time, but it may not end up as nicely shaped because you won't be able to use the vortex method.

Sweet Potato–Pulled Pork Hash

Serves 6

PREHEAT the oven to 375°F.

IN a large ovenproof skillet, heat the olive oil over medium. Add the onion and bell pepper. Sauté until soft, about 8 minutes. Add the garlic and sauté for 2 minutes more. Add the sweet potatoes, pulled pork, spinach, paprika, salt, and black pepper. Stir to combine and cook, stirring frequently, for 5 minutes. Add the beaten eggs and stir until everything is coated with egg. Press the hash down with a spatula to compact it in the skillet. Put the skillet in the oven and bake for 15 minutes, or until the sweet potatoes look crispy.

CUT into wedges and garnish with avocado, scallions, and jalapeño.

1 tablespoon olive oil

1 medium yellow onion, chopped

1 red bell pepper, chopped

2 garlic cloves, minced

5 medium sweet potatoes, grated

1½ cups pulled pork

½ cup coarsely chopped fresh spinach

1½ teaspoons smoked paprika

1 teaspoon sea salt

½ teaspoon freshly ground black pepper

3 large eggs, lightly beaten

1 avocado, cut into small cubes

3 scallions, thinly sliced

1 small jalapeño, thinly sliced

VARIATIONS

- Use shredded chicken or beef instead of pork.
- Use different colors of peppers.
- For a different flavor profile, garnish with sautéed mushrooms and onions or a drizzle of leftover marinara sauce with chopped fresh tomatoes and minced fresh basil, oregano, or thyme.

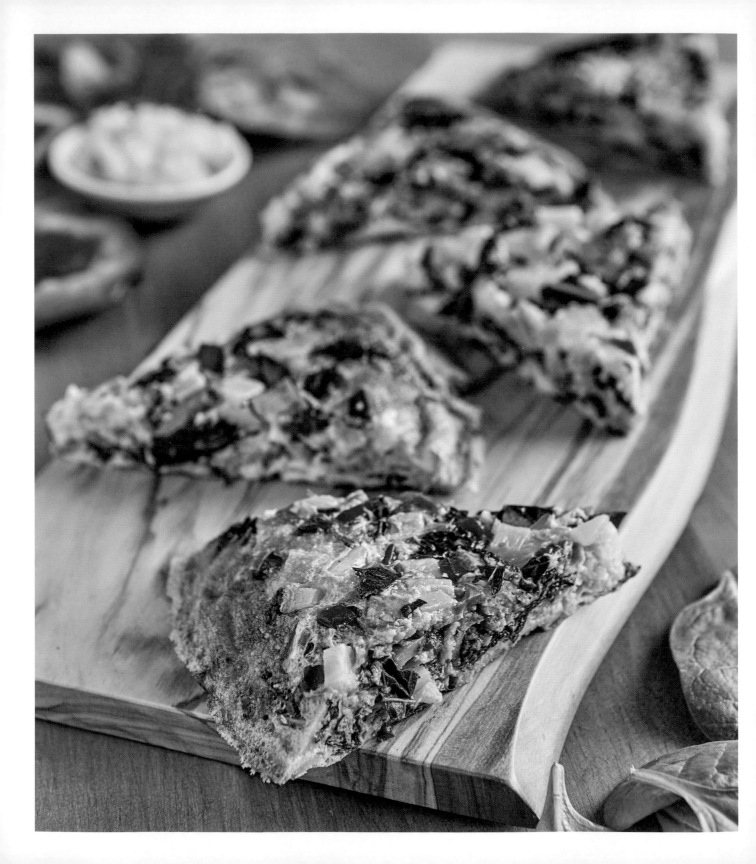

Tropical Frittata

Serves 4

PREHEAT the oven to 350°F.

IN an ovenproof skillet, melt the coconut oil over medium heat. Add the ham and sauté for 5 minutes. Add the onion and bell pepper and sauté for 5 minutes more. Add the mushrooms and sauté for 3 minutes. Add the pineapple and sauté for 3 minutes more. Add the kale and stir until wilted. Remove the pan from the heat. Sprinkle the cheese (if using) evenly over the vegetable mixture.

IN a medium bowl, whisk together the coconut milk, egg whites, eggs, baking soda, garlic powder, five-spice powder, salt, and black pepper. Pour the egg mixture evenly over the vegetable mixture. Put the skillet in the oven and bake for 30 minutes, or until the eggs are set in the middle. Remove from the oven, cut into wedges, and serve.

1 tablespoon coconut oil

8 ounces nitrate-free ham, cut into small pieces

1 sweet onion, diced

1 red bell pepper, diced

1 cup chopped mushrooms

1 cup cubed fresh pineapple (or use canned pineapple tidbits, drained)

2 cups coarsely chopped lacinato kale or fresh spinach

½ cup grated almond cheese or other dairy-free, soy-free cheese (store-bought, or make your own with the recipe on page 264; optional)

1 cup coconut milk

4 egg whites

2 large eggs

½ teaspoon baking soda

¼ teaspoon garlic powder

¼ teaspoon Chinese five-spice powder

¼ teaspoon sea salt

Dash of freshly ground black pepper

Spiced Lamb Scramble

Serves 5

IN a large skillet, combine the ground lamb, parsley, garlic, paprika, cumin, salt, cinnamon, coriander, black pepper, and cayenne (if using). Cook over medium heat, stirring frequently, until the lamb is browned. Scoop the lamb mixture into a bowl and set aside.

WITHOUT cleaning the pan, heat 1 tablespoon of the grapeseed oil in the same skillet. Add the sweet potato and shallot. Cook, stirring frequently, until the sweet potato is easily pierced with a fork. Add the broccoli and cook, stirring frequently, until it is bright green. Return the lamb mixture to the skillet and stir to fully combine everything.

PUSH everything to the edges of the pan. Pour the eggs into the middle and stir to scramble them. When they are firm, mix everything together to combine with the eggs. Serve immediately.

8 ounces ground lamb

1 tablespoon chopped fresh flat-leaf parsley

1 garlic clove, minced

½ teaspoon smoked paprika

½ teaspoon ground cumin

½ teaspoon sea salt

¼ teaspoon ground cinnamon

¼ teaspoon ground coriander

¼ teaspoon freshly ground black pepper

Dash of cayenne pepper (optional)

2 tablespoons grapeseed oil

1 large sweet potato, peeled and cut into small cubes

1 large shallot, minced

½ cup chopped broccoli

3 large eggs, lightly beaten

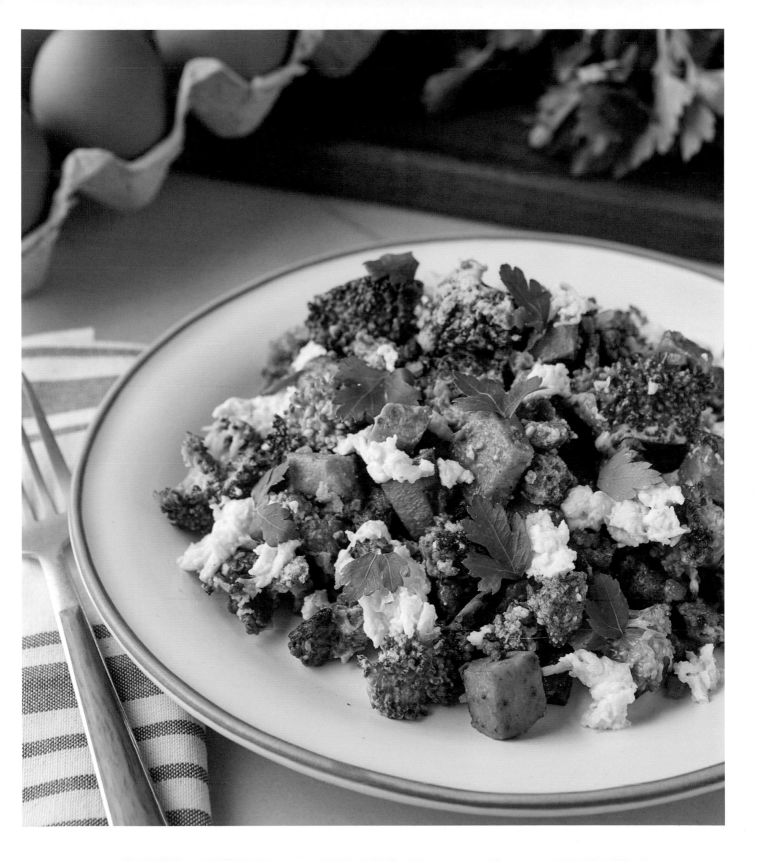

Chicken Sausage
and Vegetable Stir-Fry

Serves 4

IN a large skillet with a lid, combine the sausage and ¼ cup water. Cover the pan and bring the water to a simmer over medium-low heat. Simmer until the water cooks out, turning the sausages occasionally, about 12 minutes.

MEANWHILE, in a separate skillet or Dutch oven, heat the olive oil over medium-high heat. Add the bell peppers and sauté until they are tender, about 8 minutes. Add the broccoli and sauté, stirring frequently, until it turns bright green, about 5 minutes more. Stir in the tomatoes, seasoning, salt, and black pepper. Reduce the heat to medium-low.

CUT the sausage into ½-inch-thick slices and stir them into the vegetable mixture. Spoon into bowls and serve.

1 pound nitrate-free, no-sugar-added Italian-style chicken sausage links

2 tablespoons olive oil

2 red bell peppers, sliced

1 green bell pepper, sliced

1 small head broccoli, cut into florets

1 (14- to 15-ounce) can fire-roasted diced tomatoes

1 tablespoon Italian seasoning, or 1 teaspoon each dried oregano, basil, and thyme

½ teaspoon sea salt

¼ teaspoon freshly ground black pepper

VARIATIONS

- Use nitrate-free, no-sugar-added ground turkey sausage or strips of lean steak instead of chicken sausage links.

- Substitute any vegetables you have that you like in a stir-fry.

- If you have more time to make brown rice or quinoa, or have leftovers, you could serve this stir-fry over grains—even oatmeal.

Savory Spinach and Sausage Skillet

Serves 4

IN a large skillet, heat the oil over medium heat. Add the onion and sauté for about 5 minutes, until it starts to caramelize.

ADD the bell pepper, garlic, and red pepper flakes and sauté until the pepper slices soften.

ADD the sausage and cook, using a wooden spoon or spatula to break it up in the pan, until fully cooked through. Remove the pan from the heat. Stir in the spinach. The steam alone will lightly wilt the spinach to the perfect consistency.

SEASON with the lemon zest, lemon juice, and salt and serve.

2 tablespoons olive or coconut oil

1 sweet yellow onion, thinly sliced (about 2 cups)

1 large red bell pepper, sliced (about 2 cups)

1 garlic clove, chopped

¼ teaspoon red pepper flakes

1 pound nitrate-free, no-sugar-added mild Italian-style chicken or turkey sausage (remove casings)

5 cups baby spinach

Zest and juice of ½ lemon

Sea salt

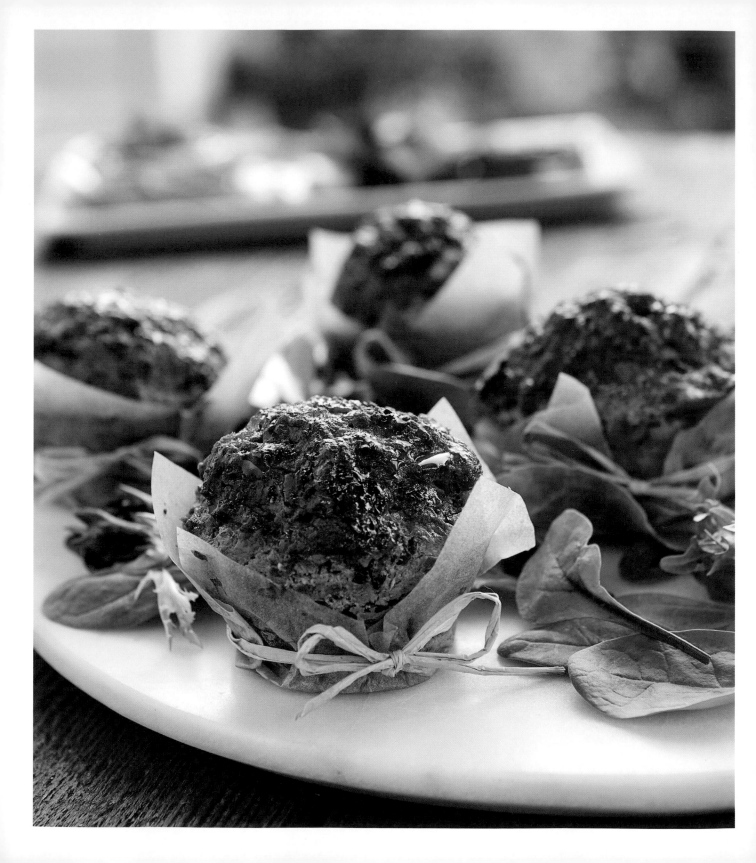

Breakfast Muffin Tin Meat Loaf

Serves 6

PREHEAT the oven to 350°F.

IN a medium nonstick skillet, heat the olive oil over medium heat. When the oil is warm, add the bell peppers and onion and sauté until just soft, about 4 minutes. Stir in the kale, remove from the heat, and set aside.

IN a large bowl, break up the ground beef, then add the bell pepper mixture, salsa, egg, paprika, chili powder, garlic powder, onion powder, cayenne, salt, and black pepper. Using your hands, mix everything together until well combined.

LINE a 6-cup muffin tin with squares of parchment paper. Pack the meat mixture into the cups. Bake for 35 minutes, or until the meat is sizzling. Remove from the oven.

FOR each serving, put 1 cup of the spring greens on a plate. Top with red onion and tomato slices, and top with a mini meat loaf. Top each meat loaf with 1 tablespoon of the salsa or hot sauce and 1 teaspoon of the cilantro.

1 tablespoon olive oil

¼ cup finely chopped green bell pepper

¼ cup finely chopped red bell pepper

¼ cup finely chopped onion

¼ cup finely chopped lacinato kale

1 pound lean ground beef

½ cup salsa

1 large egg, beaten

½ teaspoon smoked paprika

½ teaspoon chili powder

¼ teaspoon garlic powder

¼ teaspoon onion powder

⅛ teaspoon cayenne pepper

1 teaspoon sea salt

¼ teaspoon freshly ground black pepper

6 cups spring greens

Red onion slices, as much as you like

Tomato slices, as much as you like

6 tablespoons salsa or hot sauce

2 tablespoons chopped fresh cilantro leaves

Turkey Bacon–Spinach Egg Cups

Serves 6

PREHEAT the oven to 350°F. Line a standard 12-cup muffin tin with paper liners or parchment paper squares.

HEAT a medium nonstick skillet over medium-high heat. Add the broth, scallions, and garlic and cook until the scallions are tender. Stir in the spinach, salt, and pepper and cook until hot, stirring constantly, about 5 minutes. Remove from the heat and stir in the almond cheese (if using). Set aside.

CUT each slice of turkey bacon in half crosswise. Line each muffin cup with 2 bacon pieces, crisscrossed into an "X" shape. Divide the spinach mixture among the muffin cups, filling them evenly. Crack one egg into each cup and sprinkle with a little more pepper.

BAKE for about 20 minutes, or until the eggs are set (or cooked to the degree of doneness you prefer). Remove the egg cups from the pan and serve.

¼ cup chicken broth

1 cup thinly sliced scallions

3 garlic cloves, minced

2 (10-ounce) boxes frozen chopped spinach, thawed in a strainer and drained

½ teaspoon sea salt

¼ teaspoon freshly ground black pepper, plus a little for the tops of the egg cups

½ cup shredded almond cheese or other dairy-free, soy-free cheese (store-bought, or make your own with the recipe on page 264; optional)

12 slices nitrate-free, no-sugar-added turkey bacon

6 large eggs

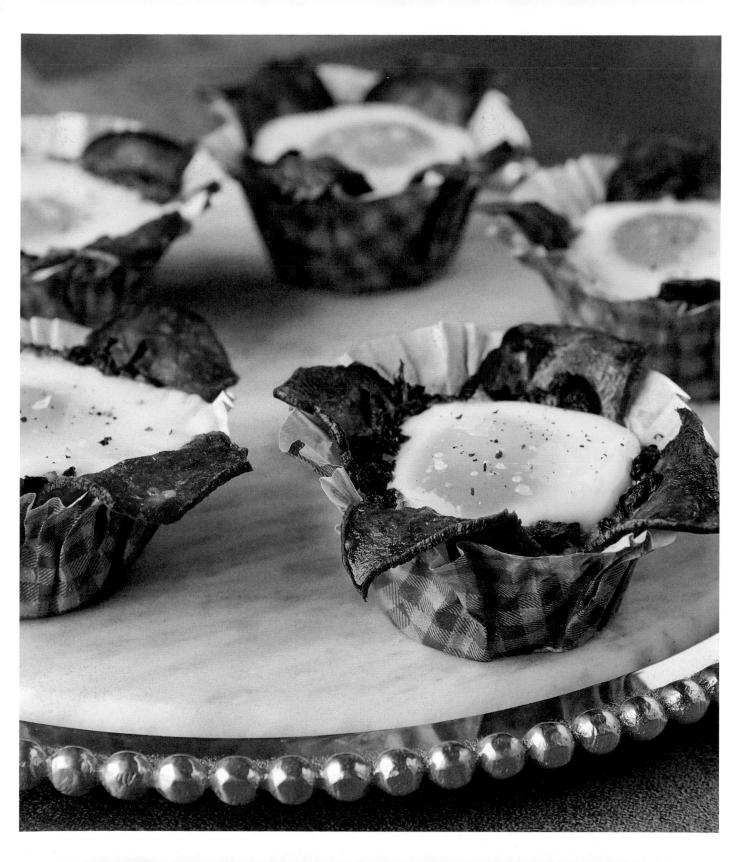

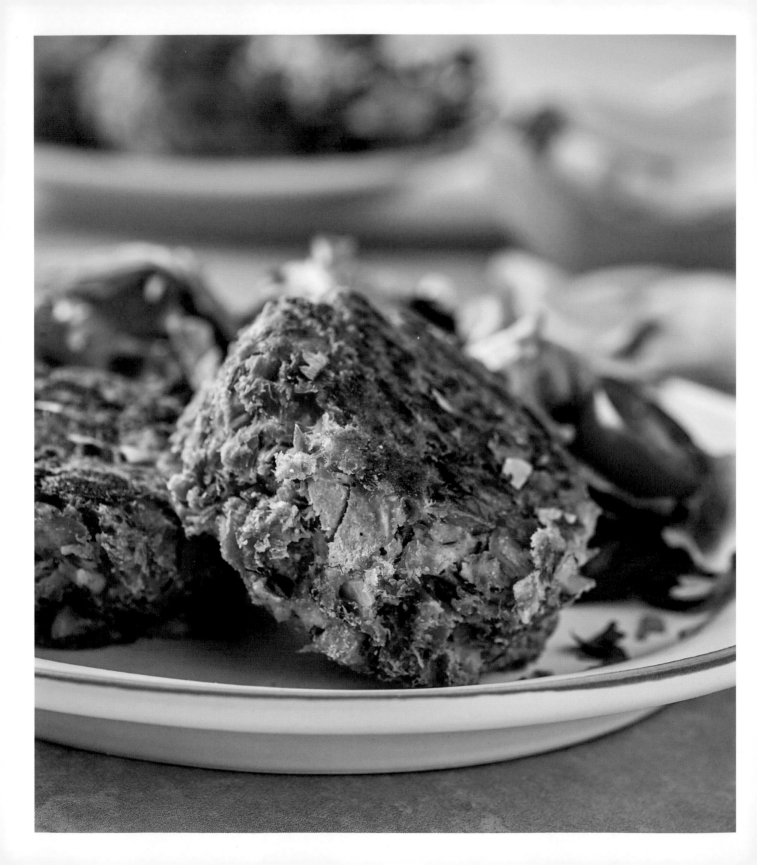

Herbed Salmon Cakes

Serves 4

PREHEAT the oven to 350°F. Line a baking sheet with parchment paper.

IN a large bowl, beat the eggs lightly. Add the salmon and break it into flakes with a fork. Add the oat flour, onion, parsley, garlic, lemon juice, mustard, thyme, salt, and pepper. Stir to fully combine.

USING your hands, form the salmon mixture into four patties. Put them on the prepared baking sheet. Bake the salmon cakes for 30 minutes, or until golden brown and starting to look crispy. Carefully flip them over halfway through the baking time.

DIVIDE the lettuce and cherry tomatoes among four plates and top each with a warm salmon cake.

2 large eggs

15 ounces cooked (or canned) salmon

½ cup oat flour

½ medium red onion, finely diced

½ cup chopped fresh flat-leaf parsley leaves

2 garlic cloves, minced

1 tablespoon fresh lemon juice

1 teaspoon Dijon mustard (no sugar added)

½ teaspoon dried thyme

½ teaspoon sea salt

¼ teaspoon freshly ground black pepper

8 cups romaine lettuce

4 cups cherry tomatoes

Cauliflower Mash Breakfast Bowl

Serves 3

FILL a saucepan with two inches of water and bring to a boil over high heat. Put the cauliflower into a steamer basket and set it over the boiling water. Cover and cook until the cauliflower is soft, about 10 minutes (you should be able to pierce it easily with a fork). Put the cauliflower in a large bowl. Add ½ teaspoon of the salt and ¼ teaspoon of the pepper, then mash with a potato masher or fork until smooth. Divide the cauliflower mash among three bowls. Set aside.

IN a medium skillet, heat the olive oil over medium heat. Add the mushrooms, bacon, garlic, and remaining ½ teaspoon salt and ¼ teaspoon pepper. Sauté until the bacon is crisp and the mushrooms shrink down and soften, about 5 minutes. Add the coconut aminos and stir to coat the mushrooms. Stir in the spinach. Cook for 2 minutes more.

DIVIDE the bacon-mushroom mixture among the bowls of cauliflower mash and serve.

½ head cauliflower, cut into florets

1 teaspoon sea salt

½ teaspoon freshly ground black pepper

1 tablespoon olive oil

2 cups cremini or baby bella mushrooms, cut in half

6 slices nitrate-free, no-sugar-added turkey bacon, chopped

1 garlic clove, minced

3 tablespoons coconut aminos

4 cups baby spinach

VARIATIONS

- Use nitrate-free, no-sugar-added ground turkey sausage instead of bacon.
- Make this with baby kale instead of spinach.
- Instead of mushrooms, you could use sautéed bell pepper strips or chopped fresh tomatoes.
- For a vegetarian version, omit the bacon and increase the mushrooms to 3 cups.

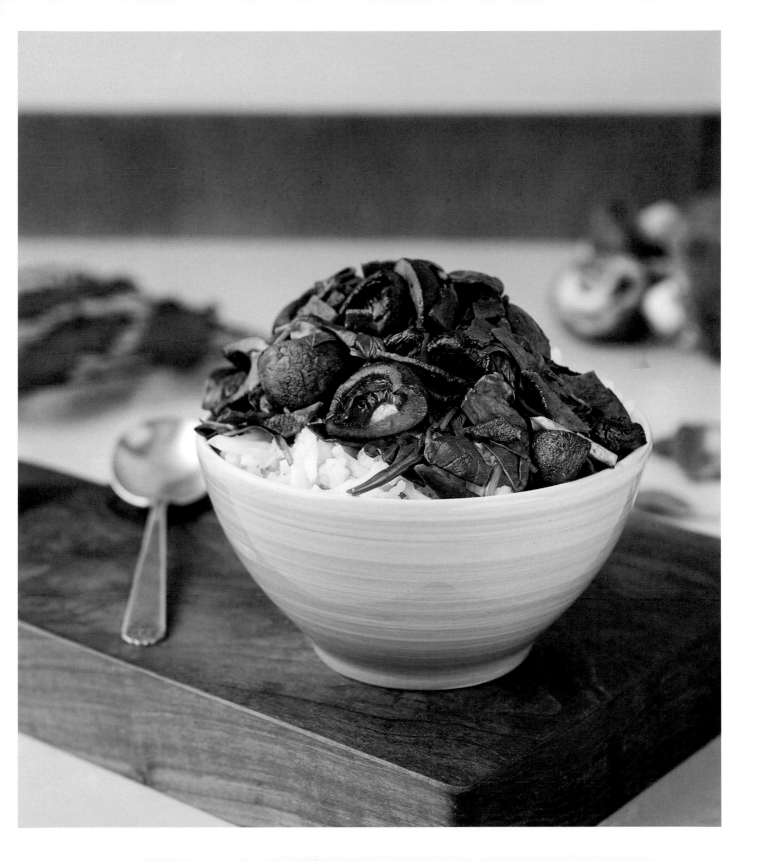

LUNCHES

Mushroom Soup

Serves 2

IN a large pot or Dutch oven, heat the olive oil over medium-high heat. Add the onions and sauté until soft, about 4 minutes. Add the mushrooms, garlic, thyme, and allspice. Mix well and cook for about 5 minutes. Add the vinegar and stir to combine. Stir in the almond flour and cook, stirring continuously, for 2 minutes. Add the broth, stir to combine everything, then bring the soup to a boil. Reduce the heat to medium-low and cover the pot. Simmer for 15 minutes. Remove the pan from the heat and stir in the coconut cream. Add the tamari, salt, and pepper. To serve, ladle into bowls and garnish each bowl with a parsley sprig.

¼ cup olive oil

2 cups diced onions

16 ounces cremini or baby bella mushrooms, sliced

4 garlic cloves, minced

½ teaspoon dried thyme

⅛ teaspoon ground allspice

¼ cup white wine vinegar

¼ cup almond flour

2 cups vegetable broth

½ cup coconut cream

1 teaspoon tamari

½ teaspoon sea salt

¼ teaspoon freshly ground black pepper

2 sprigs fresh flat-leaf parsley

VARIATIONS

- Add 1 cup shredded or chopped cooked beef or chicken for a meatier soup.
- Leave out the coconut cream and increase the vegetable broth by ½ cup for a lighter, brothier mushroom soup.
- Substitute broccoli or asparagus for the mushrooms for a different cream-soup effect.

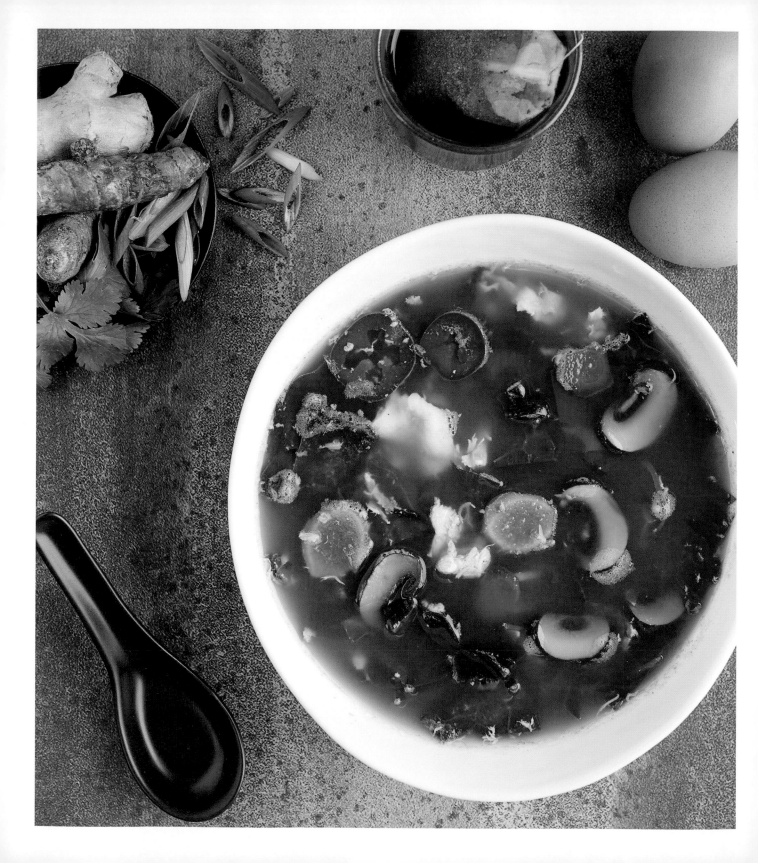

Egg Drop Soup

Serves 6

IN a large soup pot or Dutch oven, bring the broth to a simmer over medium-high heat. Add the kale, mushrooms, jalapeño, coconut aminos, turmeric, ginger, and garlic. Bring to a boil, then lower the heat to medium and simmer for 7 minutes.

MEANWHILE, in a small bowl, whisk the eggs.

UNCOVER the soup and, while stirring, slowly pour the eggs into the soup. Stir until the egg is completely cooked. Remove from the heat.

STIR in the scallions and cilantro. Season with the salt and pepper and serve.

8 cups chicken broth, vegetable broth, or bone broth

4 cups chopped fresh kale, Swiss chard, or spinach

2 cups sliced cremini or baby bella mushrooms

1 small jalapeño, sliced

2 tablespoons coconut aminos

1 tablespoon grated fresh turmeric, or 1 teaspoon ground

1 tablespoon grated fresh ginger, or 1 teaspoon ground

2 garlic cloves, minced

4 large eggs

2 medium scallions, thinly sliced

2 tablespoons chopped fresh cilantro

1 teaspoon sea salt

½ teaspoon freshly ground black pepper

Cashew Soup

Serves 6

IN a medium skillet, melt the coconut oil over medium-high heat. Add the chicken and sauté until it is browned, about 5 minutes. Add the onion and bell pepper. Sauté for 5 minutes more. Add the jalapeños, ginger, garlic, coriander, and cumin. Cook for 3 minutes, stirring to coat the vegetables with the spices. Remove the skillet from the heat.

IN a large soup pot or Dutch oven, bring the broth to a simmer over medium-high heat. Add the cashew butter and whisk until it is fully melted into the broth, about 3 minutes. Add the sweet potato and tomato. Simmer for 20 minutes. Add the chicken mixture from the skillet. Simmer for 15 minutes more. Stir in the spinach and cilantro, then remove from the heat. Season with the salt and black pepper.

DIVIDE the soup among six bowls. Divide the cashews among the bowls, sprinkling them on top of the soup, and serve.

VARIATION

- You could make this in the slow cooker. Whisk the broth and cashew butter together first, then add all the other ingredients, cover, and cook on high for 6 hours or on low for 8 to 10 hours.

1 tablespoon coconut oil

1 chicken breast, cut into ½-inch pieces

1 medium yellow onion, chopped

1 red bell pepper, cut into small cubes

2 jalapeños, seeded and minced

2 tablespoons minced fresh ginger

2 garlic cloves, minced

1 tablespoon ground coriander

2 teaspoons ground cumin

4 cups chicken broth

¾ cup cashew butter

1 large sweet potato, peeled and cut into ½-inch cubes

1 cup chopped fresh tomato

3 cups baby spinach

½ cup chopped fresh cilantro

1 teaspoon sea salt

½ teaspoon freshly ground black pepper

½ cup raw cashews, crushed or whole

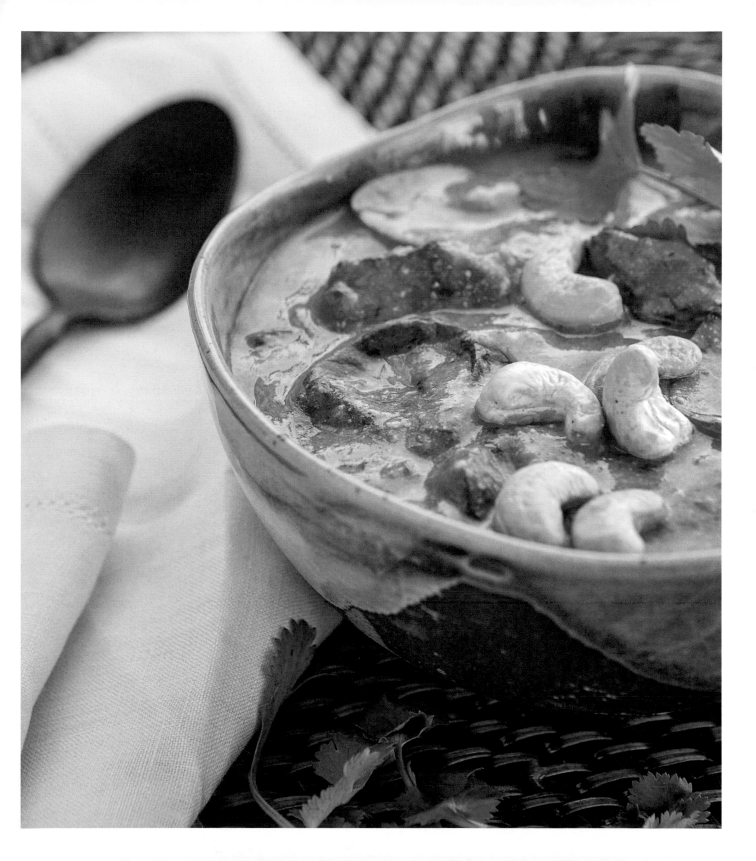

Chicken Pho

Serves 4

IN a soup pot or Dutch oven, combine the broth, onion, ginger, cinnamon stick, coconut aminos, salt, pepper, and cloves and stir to combine. Add the chicken breasts. Bring the broth to a boil over medium-high heat, then reduce the heat to medium-low and cover the pot. Simmer until the chicken is completely cooked through, about 15 minutes. Cut one of the chicken breasts in half to see if it is cooked all the way through. If it still has some pink at the center, simmer for 5 minutes more, then check again.

WHEN the chicken breasts are done, transfer them to a cutting board and slice them.

DIVIDE the zucchini noodles between two bowls and top them evenly with the chicken. Divide the scallions, chopped cilantro, and basil between the bowls, piling them on top of the chicken. Squeeze one lime quarter over each bowl.

USING a slotted spoon, remove the ginger and cinnamon stick from the broth, then ladle the hot broth into each bowl. Garnish each bowl with a sprig of cilantro and top with hot sauce, if desired.

4 cups chicken broth

1 small yellow onion, thinly sliced

1 (1-inch) piece fresh ginger, sliced

1 (3-inch) cinnamon stick

2 tablespoons coconut aminos

½ teaspoon sea salt

½ teaspoon freshly ground black pepper

Pinch of ground cloves

1 pound boneless, skinless chicken breasts

1 pound zucchini, cut into noodle shapes or "spiralized"

1 bunch scallions, thinly sliced

½ cup chopped fresh cilantro, leaves, plus 4 small sprigs for garnish

16 large fresh basil leaves, rolled up and thinly sliced crosswise

1 lime, quartered

Hot sauce, such as chili garlic sauce or sriracha (optional)

VARIATIONS

- Add 8 ounces rice noodles, cooked, to the bottom of the bowls instead of or in addition to the zucchini noodles.

- Make beef pho by using beef broth instead of chicken broth, eliminating the chicken, and putting 1 pound (total for all servings) sliced tender cooked steak over the zucchini noodles before ladling in the broth.

Steak Stew

Serves 6

IN a soup pot or Dutch oven, heat ¼ cup of the broth over medium heat. Add the onion and cook until soft, about 8 minutes, adding more broth if necessary. Add the garlic and cook for 2 minutes more. Add ¼ cup more broth and the mushrooms. Cook until the mushrooms start to shrink down. Stir in the vinegar and coconut aminos and cook for 5 minutes more.

ADD ½ cup more broth, then add the bell pepper, zucchini, celery, carrots, parsley, oregano, and thyme. Cook until the vegetables are all soft, about 10 minutes. Add the steak and the remaining 2 cups broth and stir to combine everything. Bring the stew to a simmer, then stir in the arrowroot mixture. Cook, stirring, until the stew thickens, about 10 minutes more. To serve, divide the stew among four wide, shallow bowls.

3 cups beef broth

1 yellow onion, diced

4 garlic cloves, minced

1 pound cremini or baby bella mushrooms, sliced

1 tablespoon balsamic vinegar

1 tablespoon coconut aminos

1 red bell pepper, cubed

1 medium zucchini, cubed

2 celery stalks, sliced

2 carrots, sliced

1 tablespoon chopped fresh flat-leaf parsley leaves

1 teaspoon dried oregano

½ teaspoon dried thyme

1 pound cooked steak (any type), diced

1 tablespoon arrowroot powder, mixed with 2 teaspoons water

VARIATIONS

- This recipe works with any leftover cooked meat, like chicken breasts or thighs or pork chops.
- For a vegetarian version, use mushrooms, or vegetable broth, eliminate the steak, and double the mushrooms.

Asian Sesame Slaw with Grilled Steak Strips

Serves 2

IN a wide shallow bowl, whisk together the coconut aminos, sesame oil, xylitol, vinegar, garlic, five-spice powder, and ginger. Pour about half the marinade into a separate container and reserve it for the coleslaw. Add the steak to the remaining marinade, turning it a few times to coat. Cover and marinate for 1 hour at room temperature or overnight in the refrigerator. (Take the steak out of the fridge 30 minutes before cooking so it can come to room temperature.)

IN a large skillet, heat the olive oil over medium-high heat. When the oil is hot, add the steak. Sear it on one side for 3 minutes, or until you can easily flip it. Sear it on the other side for 2 minutes. The outside should be dark and crusty but the inside should still be pink. Transfer the steak to a plate; cover and let it rest while you prepare the slaw.

IN a large bowl, combine the cabbage, quinoa, cucumber, snow peas, and the reserved marinade. Toss until the marinade coats all the vegetables. Divide the cabbage mixture between two bowls. Top each with the avocado and radishes. Thinly slice the steak and divide it between the bowls, then top with the scallions, sesame seeds, and jalapeño (if using).

¼ cup coconut aminos

1 tablespoon toasted sesame oil

1 tablespoon xylitol

1 tablespoon unseasoned rice vinegar

2 garlic cloves, minced

2 teaspoons Chinese five-spice powder

1 teaspoon minced fresh ginger, or ½ teaspoon ground

8 ounces flank steak (other cuts of steak will also work)

1 tablespoon olive oil

2 cups finely shredded cabbage

⅔ cup cooked tricolor quinoa

½ cucumber, peeled, seeded, and cut into small cubes

½ cup cooked snow peas, cut in half lengthwise

½ avocado, sliced

3 radishes, thinly sliced

2 scallions, finely chopped

1 teaspoon mixed black and white sesame seeds

1 jalapeño or serrano chile, seeded and very thinly sliced (optional)

VARIATIONS

- Use chicken strips or pork strips instead of beef.
- Use brown rice instead of quinoa.

Chef's Salad Parchment Wrap

Serves 1

ON a work surface, lay down a piece of freezer paper, parchment, or wax paper about 12 inches long. Near one corner, place the turkey slices in a single, overlapping layer. Top with the ham. Layer on the egg and veggies. Drizzle with the oil and vinegar, and season with salt and pepper. Starting from the corner, roll the paper as tightly as you can around the filling, folding in the edges burrito-style as you go. Secure with a piece of tape, if necessary. To eat, peel back the paper as you eat the wrap.

2 ounces sliced nitrate-free, no-sugar-added deli turkey

1 ounce sliced nitrate-free, no-sugar-added deli ham

½ large hard-boiled egg, sliced

2 slices tomato, or ¼ cup halved cherry tomatoes

¼ cup cucumber sticks

¼ cup carrot sticks

¼ avocado, sliced

1 radish, sliced

1¼ cups shredded romaine lettuce

2 teaspoons olive oil

1 teaspoon red wine vinegar

Sea salt

Freshly ground black pepper

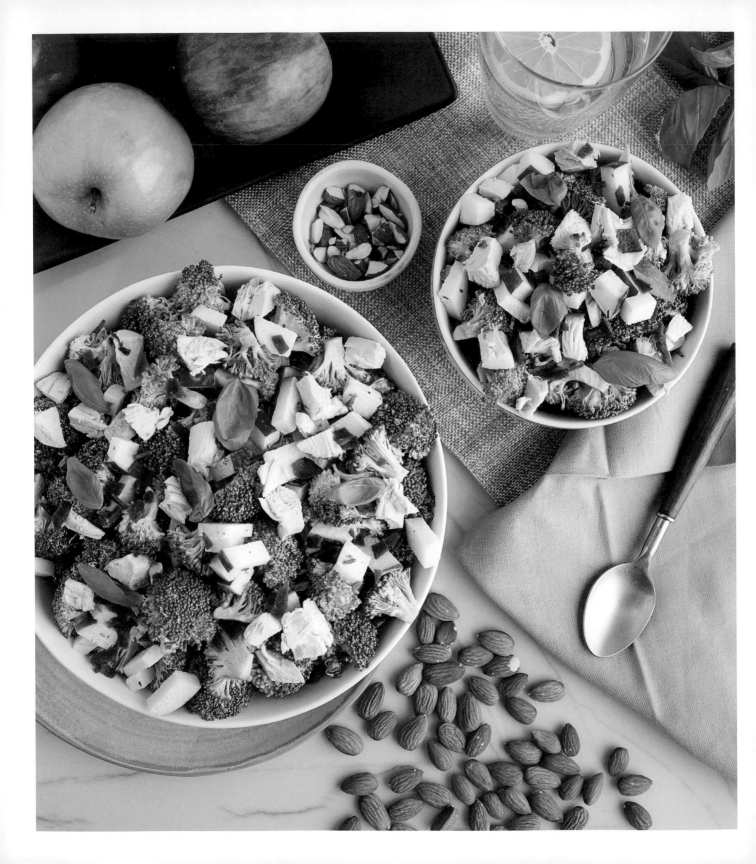

Crunchy Broccoli Apple Chicken Salad

Serves 2

MAKE the vinaigrette: In a high-powered blender, combine the mayonnaise, mustard, vinegar, rosemary, basil, garlic, lemon juice, xylitol (if using), salt, and pepper. Blend until smooth.

MAKE the salad: In a large bowl, stir together the broccoli, apples, and chicken to combine.

POUR the dressing over the salad and toss to coat everything with the dressing. This salad tastes best if you refrigerate it for at least 2 hours or up to 3 days in an airtight container before serving. Just before serving, toss in the bacon and almonds.

VARIATIONS

- Use Asian pears instead of apples.
- Try turkey instead of chicken.
- Use walnuts instead of almonds.

Vinaigrette

¼ cup safflower mayonnaise

1 tablespoon Dijon mustard (no sugar added)

1 tablespoon white wine vinegar

1 tablespoon fresh rosemary

2 fresh basil leaves

1 garlic clove, chopped

Juice of 1 lemon

¼ teaspoon xylitol (optional)

½ teaspoon sea salt

½ teaspoon freshly ground black pepper

Salad

4 cups broccoli florets

2 large apples, cored and diced (I prefer Red Delicious)

4 ounces cooked chicken, diced

4 slices nitrate-free, no-sugar-added turkey bacon, cooked until crisp and crumbled

¼ cup raw almonds, chopped

Taco Lime Shrimp Salad

Serves 2

PREHEAT the oven to 300°F.

YOU will need two sets of nested ovenproof bowls to make the tortilla bowls. Spritz the tortillas with water. Place one in each of the larger bowls, then place the smaller bowl on top. Bake for 45 minutes, then remove from the oven and carefully remove the smaller bowls. Set the tortilla bowls aside. (You can do this one day ahead; store in sealed plastic bags at room temperature.)

PREHEAT a grill or broiler (if grilling, soak wooden skewers in water while the grill heats, or use metal skewers).

IN a medium bowl, combine ¼ cup lime juice, the chipotle powder, paprika, and cumin. Add the shrimp and toss to coat. Set aside to marinate for 15 minutes.

IF grilling, thread the shrimp onto skewers. Grill or broil the shrimp for 3 to 5 minutes on each side (depending on the size of your shrimp), until no longer pink.

IN a jar, combine the remaining ¼ cup lime juice, the cilantro, olive oil, salt, and pepper. Cover the jar and shake to combine.

PUT the greens in a large bowl. Add the avocado, onion, cherry tomatoes, and jalapeño. Drizzle with the dressing and toss well. Divide the salad between two bowls and top each evenly with the shrimp.

2 spelt or sprouted-grain tortillas

½ cup fresh lime juice

1 tablespoon chipotle powder or chili powder

1½ teaspoons paprika

½ teaspoon ground cumin

12 ounces raw shrimp (any size), peeled and deveined

⅓ cup packed coarsely chopped fresh cilantro leaves

¼ cup extra-virgin olive oil

¼ teaspoon sea salt

⅛ teaspoon freshly ground black pepper

5 cups mixed greens

1 avocado, chopped

½ red onion, sliced

½ cup halved cherry tomatoes

1 jalapeño or Fresno chile, cut into rings

VARIATIONS

- Make this with chicken or beef instead of shrimp.
- Make a veggie version by eliminating the shrimp and sautéing 12 ounces sliced mushrooms in 1 tablespoon coconut or olive oil.

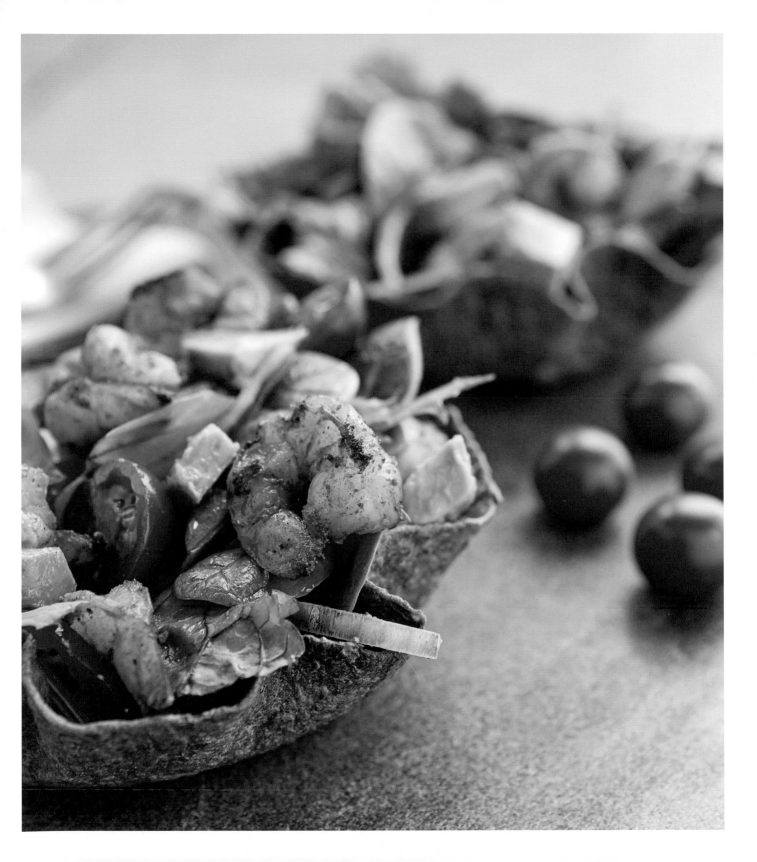

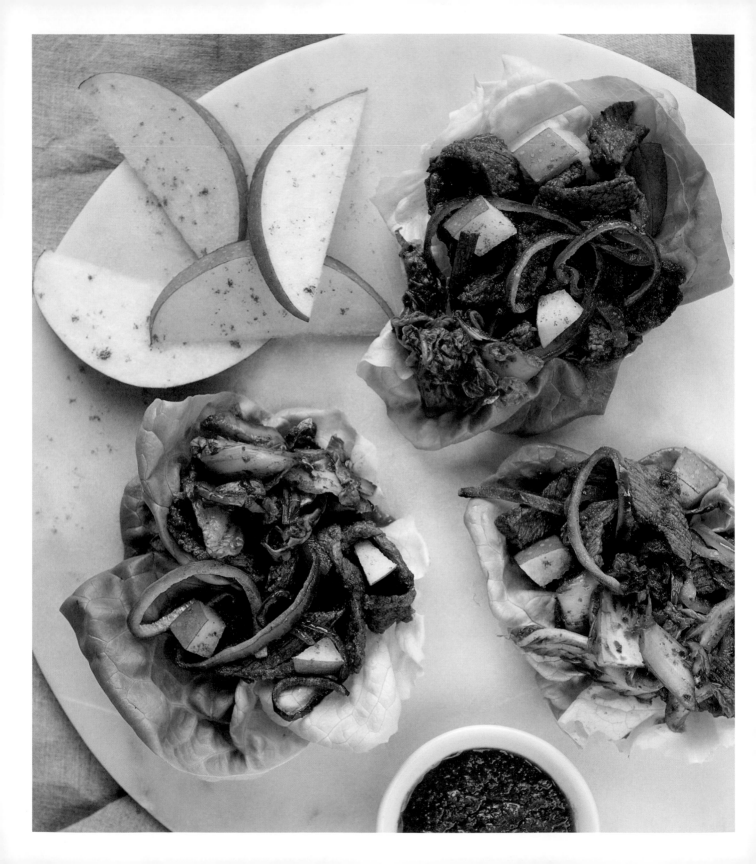

Beef Bulgogi Lettuce Cups

Serves 4

PUT the pear and water in a blender and blend until liquefied. Pour the pear puree into a bowl. Whisk in the tamari, garlic, xylitol, sesame oil, ginger, red pepper flakes, and black pepper. Add the steak strips and stir to coat the meat. Set aside at room temperature to marinate for 30 minutes.

IN a medium skillet, heat the olive oil over medium-high heat. When the oil is hot, add the onion. Sauté for 2 minutes. Add the steak and marinade. Sauté until the meat is cooked to your liking. Transfer the meat to a serving plate and drizzle it with any remaining juices from the pan. Sprinkle the scallion and sesame seeds on top.

CAREFULLY tear 8 leaves from the head of butter lettuce and arrange them on a platter. Divide the meat mixture evenly among the leaves (about 1.5 ounces per leaf) and top each with 1 tablespoon of the kimchi. Serve each person two lettuce cups.

1 Asian pear, cored and cut into pieces

½ cup water

1½ tablespoons tamari

2 garlic cloves, minced

1 tablespoon xylitol

1 teaspoon toasted sesame oil

½ teaspoon ground ginger

¼ teaspoon red pepper flakes

¼ teaspoon freshly ground black pepper

1½ pounds partially frozen ribeye, thinly sliced (freezing makes it easier to slice)

1 tablespoon olive oil

¼ small onion, thinly sliced

1 tablespoon chopped scallion

1 tablespoon sesame seeds

1 head butter lettuce

½ cup chopped kimchi

Roast Beef Rémoulade Collard Wraps

Serves 2

IN a small bowl, combine the mayonnaise, lime juice, mustard, pickle, horseradish, capers, hot sauce, salt, and pepper. Set the rémoulade aside.

POUR 2 inches of water into a large saucepan. Bring the water to a boil over high heat. Put the collard leaves in a steamer basket and set it over the boiling water. Steam the collard leaves lightly, about 3 minutes, just to make them more flexible. Divide the roast beef between the two leaves. Divide the rémoulade between the two leaves, then roll each one up, tucking in the ends. Cut each roll in half and serve.

VARIATIONS

- Use warmed sprouted-grain tortillas instead of or in addition to the collard greens.

- Try this with shrimp or tuna instead of roast beef.

- For a veggie version, substitute 1 (15-ounce) can chickpeas, drained, rinsed, and coarsely chopped, for the roast beef.

¼ cup safflower mayonnaise

Juice of ½ lime

2 tablespoons Dijon mustard (no sugar added)

1 tablespoon chopped dill pickle

2 teaspoons fresh horseradish

2 teaspoons chopped capers

1 teaspoon hot sauce

¼ teaspoon sea salt

⅛ teaspoon freshly ground black pepper

2 large collard leaves

½ pound thinly sliced roast beef

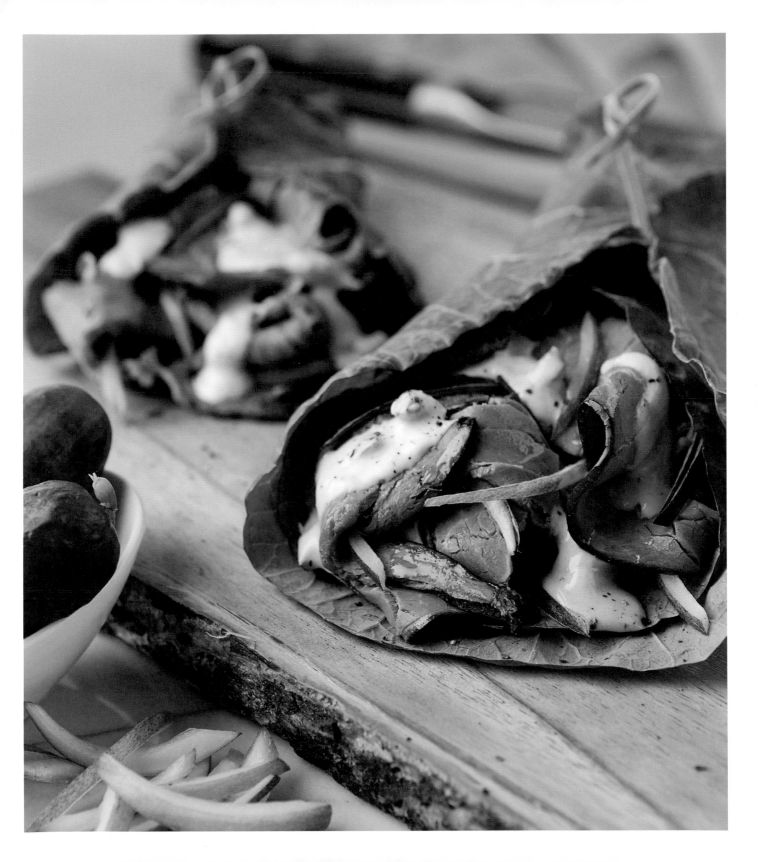

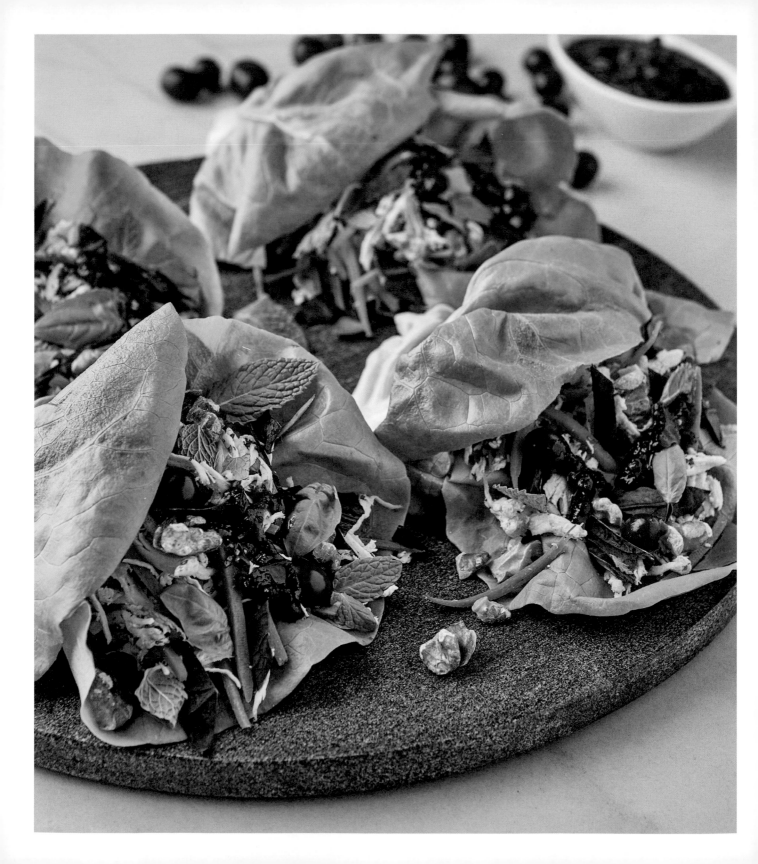

Chicken Lettuce Wraps with Cranberry Sauce

Serves 6

IN a small saucepan, combine the cranberries, water, tamari, xylitol (if using), ginger, garlic, and chile paste. Bring the mixture to a boil over medium-high heat, then lower the heat to medium-and simmer for 10 minutes. Smash the cranberries with a wooden spoon as they pop to make a sauce. (Be careful it doesn't burn, adding a little more water only if necessary—the sauce should be thick.) Remove the pan from the heat and stir in the lime zest and juice. Set aside.

IN a medium bowl, mix together the chicken, carrot, scallions, mint, basil, salt, and pepper.

LAY out the lettuce leaves and divide the chicken mixture evenly among them (you will use about 2 tablespoons per leaf). Top each mound of chicken with about 1 tablespoon of the cranberry mixture, then sprinkle the walnuts on top of each mound, dividing them evenly. Roll up the lettuce, tucking in the ends. Serve two rolls to each person.

1 cup cranberries

½ cup water

¼ cup tamari

2 tablespoons xylitol (optional)

1 tablespoon minced fresh ginger

2 garlic cloves, minced

2 teaspoons red chile paste

1 tablespoon lime zest

2 tablespoons fresh lime juice

1½ cups shredded cooked chicken breast

½ cup shredded carrot

⅓ cup thinly sliced scallions

¼ cup minced fresh mint leaves

¼ cup minced fresh basil leaves

½ teaspoon sea salt

¼ teaspoon freshly ground black pepper

12 Bibb or Boston lettuce leaves

½ cup chopped walnuts

VARIATIONS

- Make this with turkey or leftover steak instead of chicken.

- For a veggie version, use 1 (15-ounce) can white beans, drained and rinsed, in place of the chicken.

- Use sprouted-grain tortillas to wrap these up—just lay the lettuce leaves over warmed tortillas before filling.

- Eat this over leafy greens for a salad instead of a wrap.

Red Cabbage Turkey Wraps

Serves 8

IN a large bowl, combine the turkey, peaches, tomatoes, cucumber, rice, cilantro, olive oil, oregano, lemon zest, salt, hot sauce (if using), and pepper and mix thoroughly. Lay out the cabbage leaves and divide the turkey mixture among them, mounding it in the middle. Roll up the leaves, tucking in the ends, and serve.

VARIATIONS

- Use warmed sprouted-grain wraps instead of or in addition to the cabbage leaves.
- Use chicken or pork instead of turkey.
- Try a veggie version by replacing the turkey with 1 (15-ounce) can chickpeas, drained, rinsed, and coarsely chopped.

1 pound cooked turkey breast, diced, or 1 pound nitrate-free, no-sugar-added deli turkey

2 fresh peaches, pitted and diced

2 tomatoes, chopped

1 cucumber, peeled, seeded, and cut into small cubes

1 cup cooked brown rice, cooled but not refrigerated

½ cup fresh cilantro leaves

2 tablespoons extra-virgin olive oil

1 teaspoon dried oregano, crumbled

1 teaspoon lemon zest

1 teaspoon sea salt

1 teaspoon hot sauce (optional)

½ teaspoon freshly ground black pepper

8 large red cabbage leaves

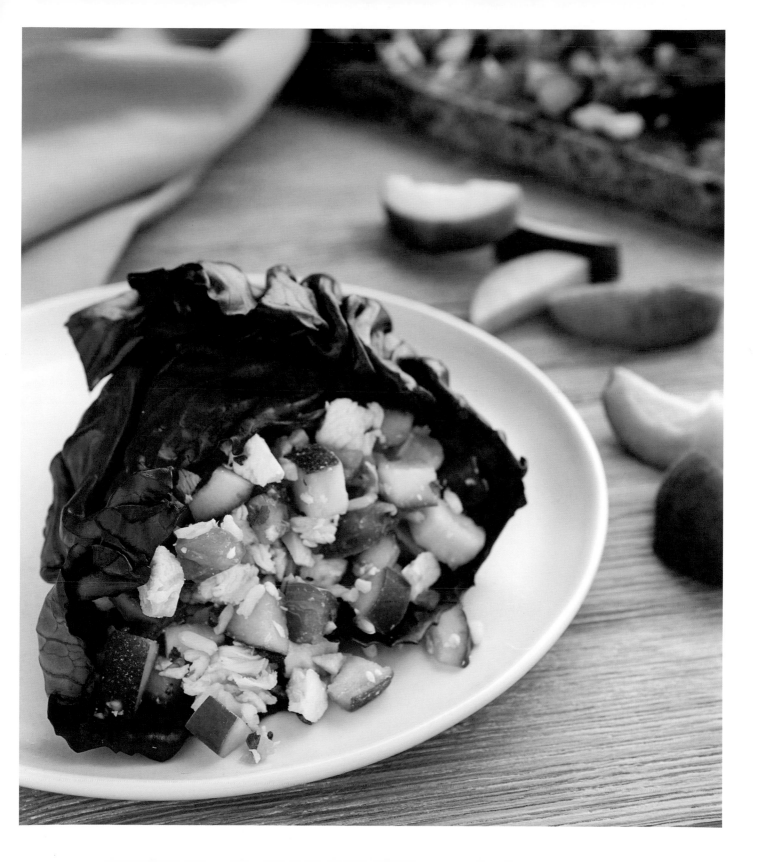

Smoky White Bean and Veggie Quesadillas

Serves 4

PUT the beans in a medium bowl and mash them with a fork until no whole beans remain. Stir in the onion, celery, mayonnaise, jalapeño, garlic powder, chili powder, ¼ teaspoon of the chipotle powder, ¼ teaspoon of the salt, the paprika, and the black pepper. Mix until everything is completely combined.

IN a large skillet, heat the olive oil over medium-high heat. Add the bell peppers and onion. Sauté until they are soft, about 8 minutes. Add the mushrooms and remaining ¼ teaspoon chipotle powder and sauté until the mushrooms shrink and everything gets very soft, about 5 minutes more. Remove from the heat and set aside.

IN a small bowl, mash the avocado with a fork. Add the lime juice and remaining ¼ teaspoon salt and mix until everything is combined.

ONE at a time, make the quesadillas: Heat a dry skillet over medium heat. Spread one-quarter of the bean mixture over half a tortilla and one-quarter of the avocado mixture over the other half. Put the tortilla in the skillet. Put the pepper mixture on top of the white bean half. When the tortilla warms up and starts to soften, fold it in half to enclose the pepper mixture. Toast the tortilla on one side for about 4 minutes. Flip the tortilla over carefully and toast the other side for about 3 minutes. Watch it closely so it doesn't burn. Transfer to a plate and repeat with the other tortillas and the remaining fillings.

1 (15-ounce) can white beans, drained and rinsed

¼ cup minced red onion

¼ cup finely chopped celery

¼ cup safflower mayonnaise

1 tablespoon minced pickled jalapeño (or a little more or less depending on how spicy you like it)

½ teaspoon garlic powder

½ teaspoon chili powder

½ teaspoon chipotle powder

½ teaspoon sea salt

¼ teaspoon smoked paprika

¼ teaspoon freshly ground black pepper

1 tablespoon olive oil

2 bell peppers, any color or a combination, cut into strips

1 white onion, thinly sliced

8 ounces white mushrooms, sliced

1 avocado, pitted

1 teaspoon fresh lime juice

4 brown rice tortillas, spelt tortillas, or sprouted-grain tortillas

2 cups baby arugula

1 cup halved cherry tomatoes

SERVE each person one tortilla, cut into wedges, topped evenly with the arugula and tomatoes.

VARIATIONS

- Use chickpeas instead of white beans.

- Use chopped turkey or chicken instead of white beans, but spread one side of the tortilla with 1 tablespoon (per tortilla) of hummus to help hold everything together.

- You could make this as a sandwich on sprouted-grain bread and toast it in the skillet or a panini press.

Grilled Almond Butter and Pear Sandwich

Serves 1

HEAT a nonstick skillet over medium heat. Spread the coconut oil on one side of the bread. Place it in the skillet, oiled-side down. Grill until golden brown. Remove the skillet from the heat.

PLACE the grilled bread on a plate and cut it in half. Spread the ungrilled sides with the almond butter and sandwich the pears in between. Serve with celery and/or jicama sticks on the side.

1½ teaspoons coconut oil

1 slice sprouted-grain bread

1½ tablespoons almond butter

1 cup sliced ripe pear

Celery and/or jicama sticks

Open-Faced Jicama Steak Sandwiches

Serves 4

PREHEAT a grill or broiler.

IN a small bowl, combine the onion remaining [1/4] cup and [8/9]vinegar and set aside.

SEASON the steak with salt and pepper. Grill or broil the steak, turning it once, until medium-rare, about 12 minutes total. Let the top steak rest on a cutting board for 5 minutes, then slice.

PUT the jicama slices in a toaster oven and toast for two cycles, or until they are warm and lightly browned.

LAY one jicama slice on each of four plates and spread mustard over the jicama. Top evenly with the tomatoes, onions, steak, and arugula and serve.

1 cup thinly sliced red onion

2 teaspoons red wine vinegar

1 pound sirloin steak, about 1¼ inches thick

Sea salt

Freshly ground black pepper

4 (¼-inch-thick) slices jicama, peeled

Dijon mustard (no sugar added)

2 tomatoes, sliced

4 cups arugula

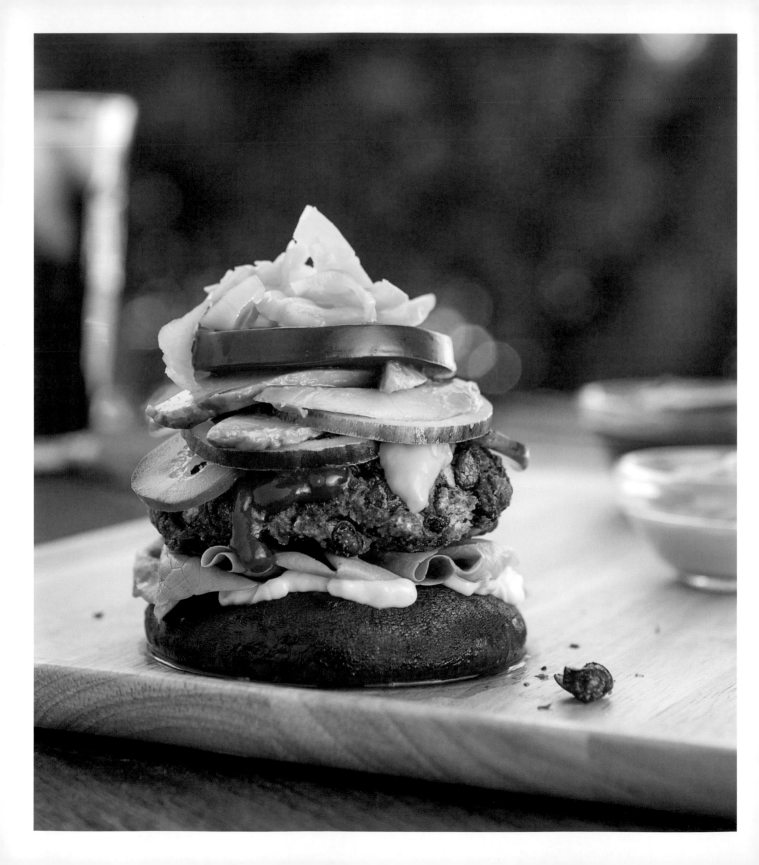

Portobello Black Bean Burgers

Serves 4

PREHEAT the oven to 375°F. Line a rimmed baking sheet with parchment paper.

MAKE the "buns": Put the mushroom caps on the prepared baking sheet, stemmed-side down. Brush the tops with the melted coconut oil and sprinkle with the salt. Bake the mushrooms for 15 minutes, or until they are soft and dark. Remove them from the oven (keep the oven on) and press them between layers of paper towels to remove excess liquid. Set aside on a plate and line the baking sheet with fresh parchment paper.

MAKE the burgers: Drain and rinse the black beans. Dry them with a paper towel, then put them in a large bowl and mash them with a fork until no whole beans remain. Mix in the zucchini, bell pepper, onion, garlic, paprika, cumin, salt, black pepper, and red pepper flakes. Stir in the bread crumbs and egg. Mix until everything is well combined.

FORM the bean mixture into four patties and put them on the prepared baking sheet. Bake the burgers for 30 minutes, or until they just start to get crispy, flipping them carefully halfway through.

TO serve, put one burger on each mushroom cap "bun" and add your desired toppings and condiments.

(continued)

"Buns"

4 large portobello mushroom caps

1 tablespoon coconut oil, melted

Pinch of sea salt

Burgers

1 (15-ounce) can black beans

1 small zucchini, shredded and pressed in colander to reduce liquid

½ green bell pepper, finely chopped

½ small onion, finely chopped

2 garlic cloves, minced

2 teaspoons smoked paprika

1 teaspoon ground cumin

½ teaspoon sea salt

½ teaspoon freshly ground black pepper

Dash of red pepper flakes

⅔ cup sprouted-grain bread crumbs

1 large egg, beaten

Portobello Black Bean Burgers (continued)

Optional toppings and condiments

Tomato slices

Lettuce leaves

Thinly sliced red onion rings

Peperoncinis

Pickles

Avocado slices

No-sugar-added ketchup

Dijon mustard (no sugar added)

Safflower mayonnaise

VARIATIONS

- Kidney beans work in this recipe as a replacement for the black beans.

- For a meaty version, use 1 pound ground turkey in place of the beans.

Salsa Penne

Serves 6

IN a large skillet, heat the olive oil over medium heat. Add the sausage, onion, bell pepper, and zucchini and sauté until the veggies are tender, about 8 minutes. Stir in the salsa, black beans, and tomatoes. Bring the mixture to a simmer and cook for about 5 minutes, or until fully heated through. Mix in the penne and serve.

1 tablespoon olive oil

12 ounces nitrate-free, no-sugar-added andouille chicken sausage

1 medium onion, diced

1 green bell pepper, chopped

1 medium zucchini, cubed

2 cups salsa

1 (15-ounce) can black beans, drained and rinsed

1 (14.5-ounce) can diced tomatoes

6 cups cooked brown rice penne

Sweet Potato Turkey Burger Sliders

Serves 4

PREHEAT the oven to 375°F. Line a large rimmed baking sheet with parchment paper.

ARRANGE the sweet potato slices in a single layer on the prepared baking sheet. Bake for 20 minutes, or until they just start to brown and you can pierce them easily with a fork, flipping them carefully after 10 minutes.

MEANWHILE, preheat a grill or broiler.

IN a medium bowl, combine the ground turkey, scallions, garlic, oats, salt, and pepper. Mix everything together with your hands, then shape the mixture into eight small patties. Brush the grill grates or a broiler pan with the olive oil and grill or broil the patties for 5 minutes on each side.

MAKE the aioli: In a blender, combine all the ingredients for the aioli. Blend until smooth. Use immediately.

TO serve, spread the aioli on each sweet potato slice. Top each slice with a turkey burger and any additional toppings you like. Serve open-faced.

1 large sweet potato, peeled, cut into four ¼-inch-thick rounds from the center (use the rest of the sweet potato for another meal)

1 pound ground turkey

2 scallions, thinly sliced

1 garlic clove, minced

2 tablespoons quick-cooking oats

½ teaspoon sea salt

¼ teaspoon freshly ground black pepper

1 teaspoon olive oil

Garlic Avocado Aioli

1 large avocado

¼ cup safflower mayonnaise

1 garlic clove, pressed through a garlic press

2 teaspoons fresh lemon juice

½ teaspoon sea salt, or to taste

Optional toppings

Tomato slices

Lettuce leaves

Thinly sliced red onion rings

Pickles

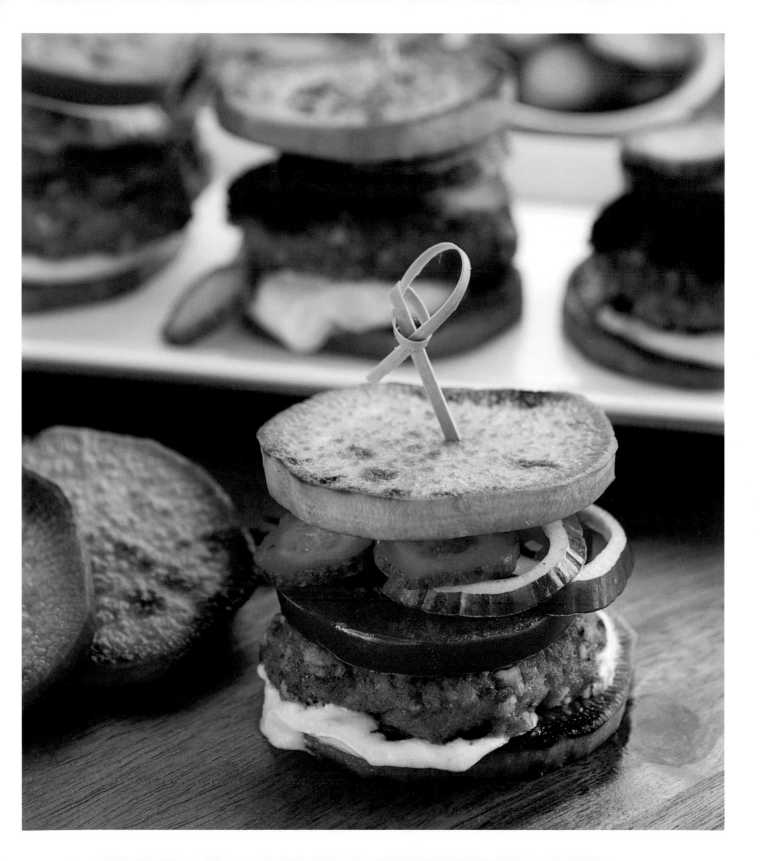

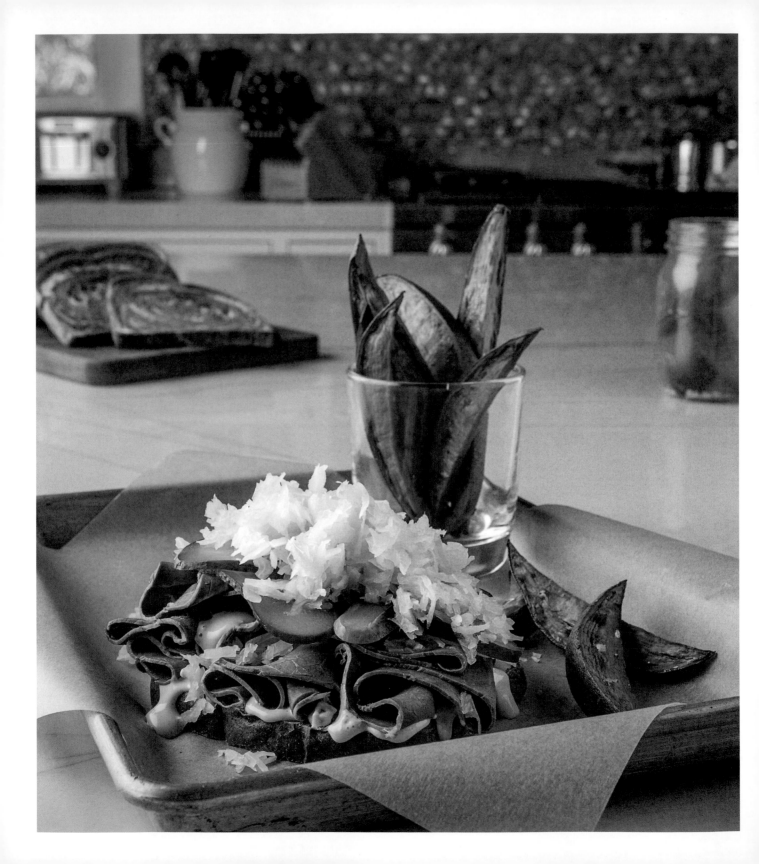

Open-Faced Reuben

Serves 2

MAKE the dressing: In a small bowl, stir together all the dressing ingredients. Cover and chill for at least 30 minutes or up to overnight before serving.

MAKE the sweet potatoes: Preheat the oven to 400°F. Line a baking sheet with parchment paper.

CUT the sweet potato into fry shapes. In a large bowl, toss the sweet potatoes with the olive oil, salt, and pepper. Spread out the sweet potatoes in a single layer on the prepared baking sheet and bake for 30 minutes, or until they start to brown and look crispy.

MEANWHILE, make the sandwiches: Put the corned beef and sauerkraut in two small baking pans, casserole dishes, or ramekins. Put them in the oven with the fries during the last 10 minutes, to warm them.

TOAST the bread. Spread each piece of toasted bread with about ¼ cup of the dressing. Take the corned beef and sauerkraut out of the oven. Divide the corned beef between the two slices of bread. Add the pickles (or serve them on the side). Top with the sauerkraut. Serve with the sweet potato fries on the side.

Dressing

½ cup safflower mayonnaise

3 tablespoons finely chopped dill pickle

2 tablespoons no-sugar-added ketchup, or 2 teaspoons tomato paste

1 tablespoon finely chopped sweet onion

1 tablespoon fresh lemon juice

⅛ teaspoon sea salt

⅛ teaspoon freshly ground black pepper

Sweet Potato Fries

1 large sweet potato

1 tablespoon olive oil

½ teaspoon sea salt

¼ teaspoon freshly ground black pepper

Sandwiches

8 ounces nitrate-free no-sugar-added corned beef

1 cup fermented sauerkraut, drained

2 slices sprouted-grain bread

2 no-sugar-added dill pickles, thinly sliced (or leave them whole and serve them on the side)

Roasted Chickpea Quinoa Buddha Bowl

Serves 2

PREHEAT the oven to 400°F. Line a rimmed baking sheet with parchment paper.

IN a small bowl, mix together the salt, oregano, black pepper, onion powder, and garlic powder. Add the chickpeas and drizzle with the olive oil, then toss to coat the chickpeas with the oil and spices. Spread the chickpeas out on the prepared baking sheet and bake for 30 minutes, stirring halfway through.

DIVIDE the greens between two bowls. Divide the quinoa between the bowls, putting it on top of the lettuce. Next, add the cucumbers, bell pepper, tomatoes, and olives, dividing them evenly. Top with the chickpeas, then scoop 2 tablespoons of the hummus on top of each bowl. Sprinkle the hummus with the paprika and serve.

1 teaspoon sea salt

½ teaspoon dried oregano

¼ teaspoon freshly ground black pepper

¼ teaspoon onion powder

¼ teaspoon garlic powder

1 cup chickpeas, drained, rinsed, and dried, skins discarded

1 teaspoon olive oil

2 cups mixed greens or chopped romaine lettuce

1 cup cooked tricolor (or any color) quinoa

2 cucumbers, peeled, seeded, and cut into small cubes

1 yellow bell pepper, cut into small cubes

1 cup grape tomatoes, halved

¼ cup pitted kalamata olives

4 tablespoons hummus

Pinch of smoked paprika

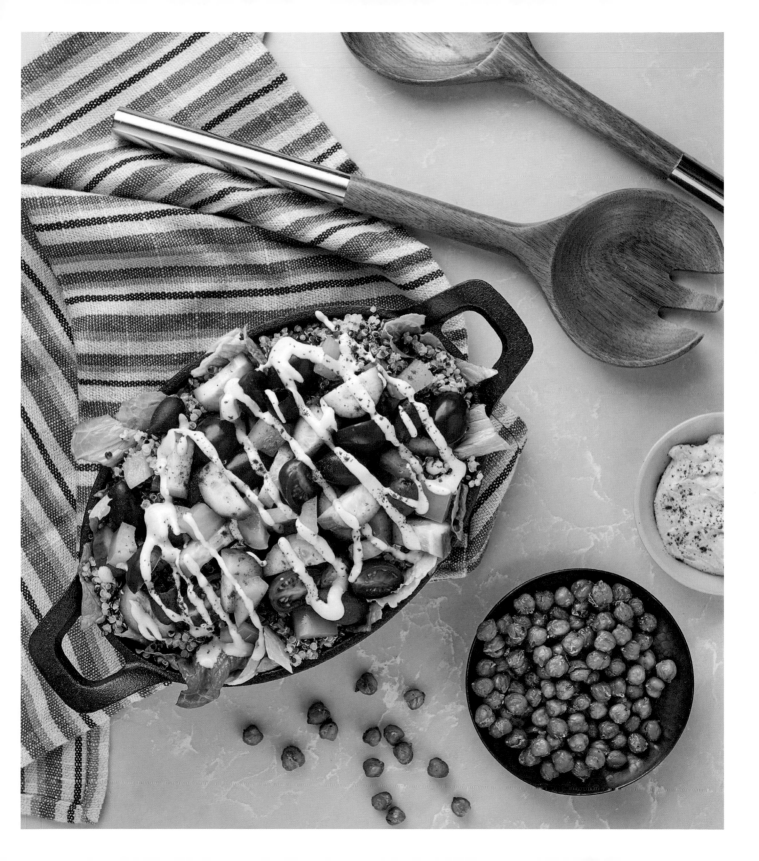

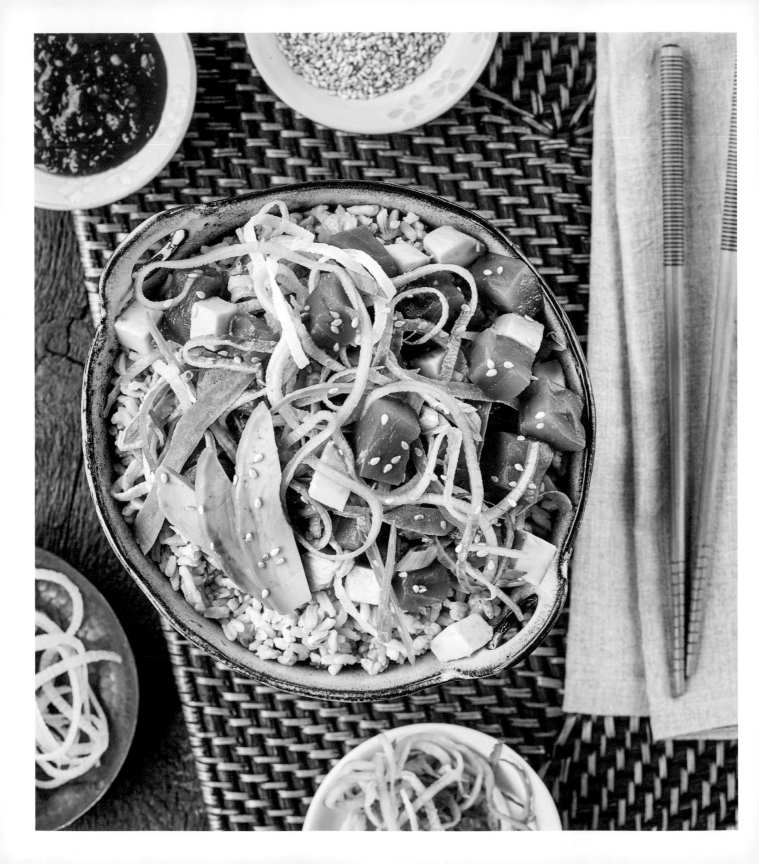

Spicy Tuna Brown Rice Poke Bowl

Serves 4

IN a medium bowl, whisk together the coconut aminos, ginger, sriracha, vinegar, sesame oil, and sesame seeds. Add the tuna and stir to coat with the marinade. Cover and refrigerate for 20 minutes.

IN a medium bowl, stir together the mayo and red chile paste. Add the tuna and marinade to the mayonnaise mixture and stir to coat the tuna. Cover and refrigerate for 15 minutes.

TO serve, put 1 cup of the rice in each bowl. Layer the daikon, cucumbers, carrots, snow peas, and avocado in each bowl. Scoop the tuna from the bowl with a slotted spoon and divide it among the bowls. Drizzle with the marinade remaining in the bowl, and top with the scallions.

VARIATION

- If raw fish isn't your thing, or if you just want to try something different, you can substitute 1 pound chicken or pork, marinated and then sautéed until cooked through, for the tuna.

¼ cup coconut aminos

2 tablespoons minced fresh ginger

1 tablespoon sriracha or chili garlic sauce

1 tablespoon unseasoned rice vinegar

1 tablespoon toasted sesame oil

I tablespoon toasted sesame seeds

24 ounces sashimi-grade raw tuna, cubed

¼ cup avocado mayo or safflower mayo

1 to 2 tablespoons red chile paste

4 cups cooked brown rice, cooled but not refrigerated

½ medium daikon radish, spiralized

4 mini cucumbers, spiralized

1 carrot, cut into ribbons with a vegetable peeler

12 snow peas

1 avocado, cut into small cubes

2 scallions, thinly sliced

Lentil Veggie Power Bowl

Serves 6

RINSE the lentils in a strainer and put them in a medium saucepan. Add the broth. Cover and bring to a boil over medium-high heat. Immediately lower the heat to medium and simmer, uncovered, for 20 minutes, or until the lentils are cooked through but still chewy. Drain them in a strainer, then put them in a large bowl.

IN a large skillet, heat the olive oil over medium-high heat. Add the onion and sauté until soft, about 5 minutes. Add the garlic and sauté for 2 minutes more. Add the bell pepper and sauté for 8 minutes more. Stir in the tomatoes, then transfer the vegetable mixture to the bowl with the lentils. While the mixture is still hot, add the spinach, parsley, salt, and black pepper and toss to combine everything.

MAKE the dressing: In a blender, combine all the ingredients for the dressing and blend until smooth.

DRIZZLE the dressing over the lentil mixture. Toss to coat everything in the dressing. Top with the scallions and serve warm or cold.

1 cup dried lentils

3 cups vegetable broth or chicken broth

1 tablespoon olive oil

1 medium red onion, chopped

3 garlic cloves, minced

1 red bell pepper, chopped

1 cup grape tomatoes, halved

2 packed cups baby spinach, coarsely chopped

¼ cup fresh parsley leaves, minced

1 teaspoon sea salt

1 teaspoon freshly ground black pepper

Lemon-Tahini Dressing

¼ cup fresh lemon juice

2 tablespoons tahini

2 tablespoons nutritional yeast

2 tablespoons extra-virgin olive oil

1 garlic clove, minced

½ teaspoon sea salt

6 tablespoons thinly sliced scallions, for serving

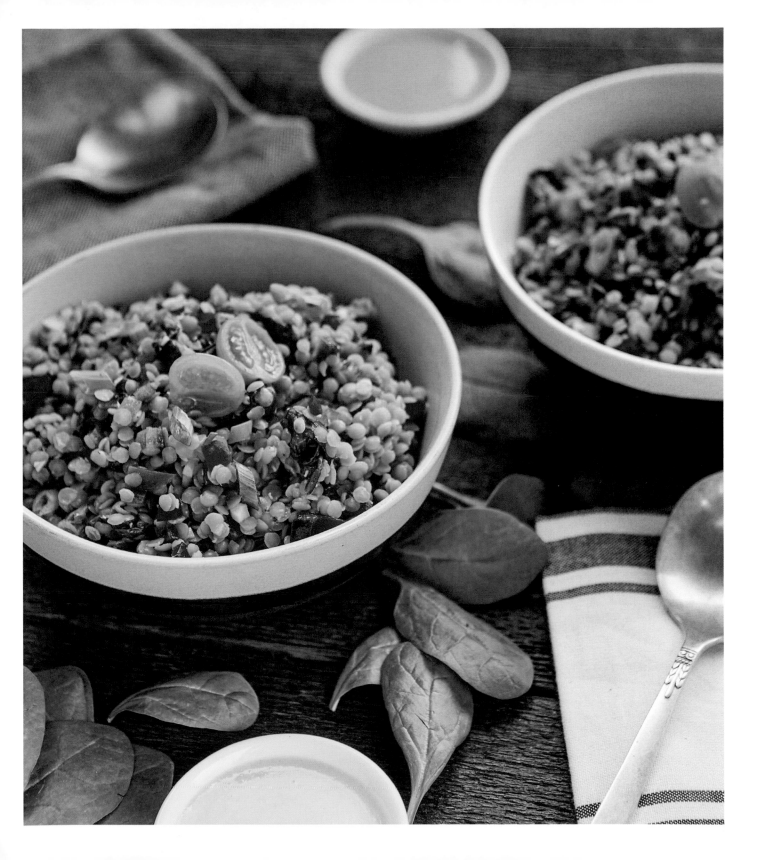

Cuban Chicken and Black Bean Quinoa Bowl

Serves 4

MAKE the sweet potatoes: Preheat the oven to 425°F. Line a baking sheet with parchment paper.

IN a large bowl, toss the sweet potatoes with the arrowroot powder and salt, then add the melted coconut oil and toss to coat. Arrange the sweet potatoes in a single layer on the prepared baking sheet. Bake for 30 to 40 minutes, stirring occasionally, until lightly browned at the edges.

MARINATE the chicken: In a blender, combine the orange puree, lime zest, lime juice, cilantro, chile, garlic, cumin, tamari, stevia, and a couple of grinds of black pepper. Blend until smooth.

PLACE the chicken in a bowl and pour ⅓ cup of the marinade over the chicken; set the remaining marinade aside. Cover the bowl and marinate the chicken for at least 20 minutes (or overnight) in the refrigerator.

MAKE the salsa: Combine the salsa ingredients in a bowl. Set aside.

MAKE the quinoa and beans: Heat a large skillet with a lid over medium-high heat. Add 2 tablespoons of the olive oil and the onions. Cook, stirring occasionally, for 5 minutes. Add the bell peppers and quinoa. Sauté for 5 minutes, until the red bell pepper is soft and the quinoa is lightly toasted. Add the broth. Bring to a boil, reduce the heat to low, cover, and simmer for 15 to 20 minutes, until the quinoa is cooked. Season with salt and black pepper and remove to a bowl or plate. Add the remaining 1 teaspoon olive oil, the garlic, black beans, and a pinch

Sweet Potatoes

2 medium sweet potatoes, cubed

1 tablespoon arrowroot powder

¼ teaspoon sea salt

2 tablespoons coconut oil, melted

Chicken and Marinade

1 orange, peeled, seeded, and pureed

1 tablespoon lime zest

½ cup fresh lime juice

3 tablespoons fresh cilantro, chopped

1 tablespoon minced fresh hot red chile

2 garlic cloves

1 teaspoon ground cumin

1 teaspoon tamari

3 or 4 drops stevia

Freshly ground black pepper

½ pound boneless, skinless chicken breast, cut into bite-size pieces

1 tablespoon olive oil

Mango Salsa

1 mango, pitted, peeled, and diced

1 fresh hot red chile, seeded and minced

¼ cup fresh cilantro, chopped

Juice of ½ lime

Quinoa and Beans

2 tablespoons plus 1 teaspoon olive oil

2 cups chopped onions

2 cups chopped red bell peppers

¾ cup dry quinoa

1½ cups chicken broth

Sea salt and freshly ground black pepper

1 garlic clove, minced

1 cup canned black beans, drained and rinsed

Sauce

1 orange, peeled, seeded, and pureed

⅓ cup full-fat canned coconut milk

each of salt and black pepper. Cook until the beans are warmed through. Cover and set aside to keep warm.

COOK the chicken: Remove the chicken from the marinade and pat dry with paper towels. In a large skillet, heat the olive oil over medium-high heat. Add the chicken and cook for 5 minutes, or until browned all over and cooked through. Remove the chicken from the pan and cover to keep warm.

ADD the reserved marinade and the orange puree to the skillet. Bring to a boil, scraping up the browned bits from the bottom of the pan. Add the coconut milk and cook for about 5 minutes, until the sauce is thick enough to coat the back of a spoon.

TO serve, divide the quinoa, black beans, chicken, sweet potatoes, and salsa evenly among four bowls. Drizzle with the sauce and serve.

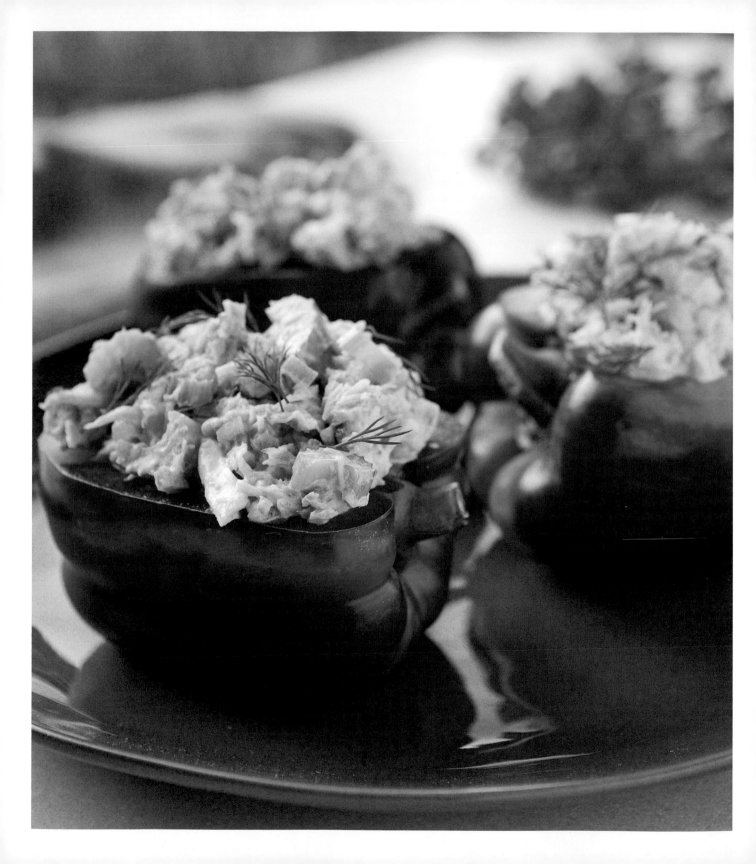

Crab-Stuffed Bell Peppers

Serves 6

IN a medium bowl, stir together the crab and mayonnaise until combined. Add the celery, parsley, shallot, lemon juice, salt, black pepper, and dill. Stuff the crab mixture into the peppers and top with the lemon zest.

VARIATION
- Try this with tuna instead of crab.

12 ounces lump crabmeat

⅓ cup safflower mayonnaise

3 celery stalks, sliced

½ cup chopped fresh parsley leaves

1 shallot, minced

Zest and juice of 1 lemon

1 teaspoon sea salt

½ teaspoon freshly ground black pepper

½ teaspoon dried dill

6 medium bell peppers (any color), tops cut off, seeds removed

Ham-Loaded Yam

Serves 2

PREHEAT the oven to 400°F. Poke holes in the yams with a fork or knife and put them directly on the oven rack. Bake until soft.

MAKE a slice lengthwise along the top of each yam and mash the flesh slightly with a fork. Top each yam with half the ham. In a medium bowl, toss together the lettuce, tomatoes, peperoncinis, olive oil, salt, oregano, and thyme. Top the ham with the salad mixture and serve.

VARIATIONS

- Top each serving with 1 or 2 tablespoons Creamy Ranch Dressing (recipe on page 270).
- You could make this with deli turkey, chicken, or roast beef instead of ham.

2 yams or sweet potatoes

½ pound nitrate-free, no-sugar-added deli ham, cut into small cubes

2 cups shredded romaine lettuce

1 cup grape tomatoes, halved (quarter larger ones)

2 peperoncinis, seeded and thinly sliced

2 teaspoons extra-virgin olive oil

½ teaspoon sea salt

½ teaspoon dried oregano

½ teaspoon dried thyme

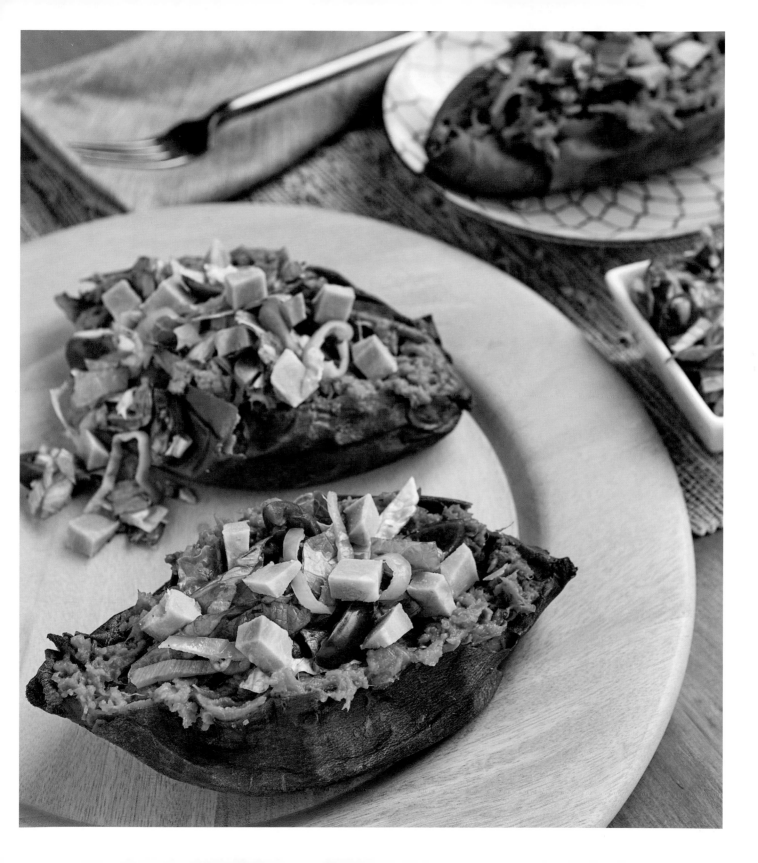

Vegan Jalapeño Popper Mac and Cashew Cheese–Stuffed Portobello Mushrooms

Serves 4

NOTE: The night before preparing this recipe, put the cashews in a jar to soak. Drain before using them.

PUT the bread in a blender and pulse until broken down into crumbs. Transfer the crumbs to a small bowl and stir in 1 tablespoon of the olive oil, ¼ teaspoon of the salt, ¼ teaspoon of the pepper, and the garlic powder. Set aside.

IN the blender, combine the cashews, water, nutritional yeast, mustard, ½ teaspoon of the salt, and ½ teaspoon of the pepper and blend until smooth and creamy. Set aside.

COOK the pasta according to the package directions. Reserve ½ cup of the pasta water, then drain the pasta. Set aside.

PREHEAT the oven to 375°F. Line a baking sheet with parchment paper.

PLACE the mushroom caps stemmed-side down on the prepared baking sheet and bake for 15 minutes. Remove the pan from the oven but leave the oven on.

IN a large nonstick skillet, heat 1 tablespoon of the olive oil over medium heat. Add the sliced onions and the remaining ¼ teaspoon each salt and pepper. Cook, stirring often, until the onions are browned, about 10 minutes. Add the spinach and stir

1 slice sprouted-grain bread, torn into pieces

3 tablespoons olive oil

1 teaspoon sea salt

1 teaspoon freshly ground black pepper

⅛ teaspoon garlic powder

½ cup raw cashews, soaked in water overnight, then drained

1½ cups water

2 tablespoons nutritional yeast

2 teaspoons Dijon mustard (no sugar added)

3 ounces brown rice pasta (or other pasta made without wheat or corn)

8 portobello mushroom caps

2 cups sliced onions, plus 1 small onion, finely chopped

5 cups baby spinach

3 garlic cloves, minced

2 jalapeños, seeded and finely chopped, plus more for serving

2 tablespoons Cashew Cream Cheese (recipe on page 266)

until it wilts completely, 2 to 3 minutes. Scrape the contents of the skillet into a bowl and set aside.

RETURN the skillet to the heat. Add the remaining 1 tablespoon olive oil and the chopped onion. Sauté for 2 minutes. Add the garlic and jalapeños and sauté for 1 minute more.

ADD the cashew sauce and cream cheese to the pan, stirring to combine. Stir in the cooked pasta and the reserved ½ cup pasta water. Cook for 2 to 3 minutes, until thick and creamy. Remove from the heat.

POUR away any mushroom liquid that has collected on the baking sheet and turn the mushroom caps gill-side up. Divide the sautéed spinach mixture evenly among the mushroom caps. Top with the pasta mixture and then the bread crumb topping. Bake for 10 minutes, until warmed through and golden brown. Serve with extra chopped jalapeños alongside, for those who like an extra kick.

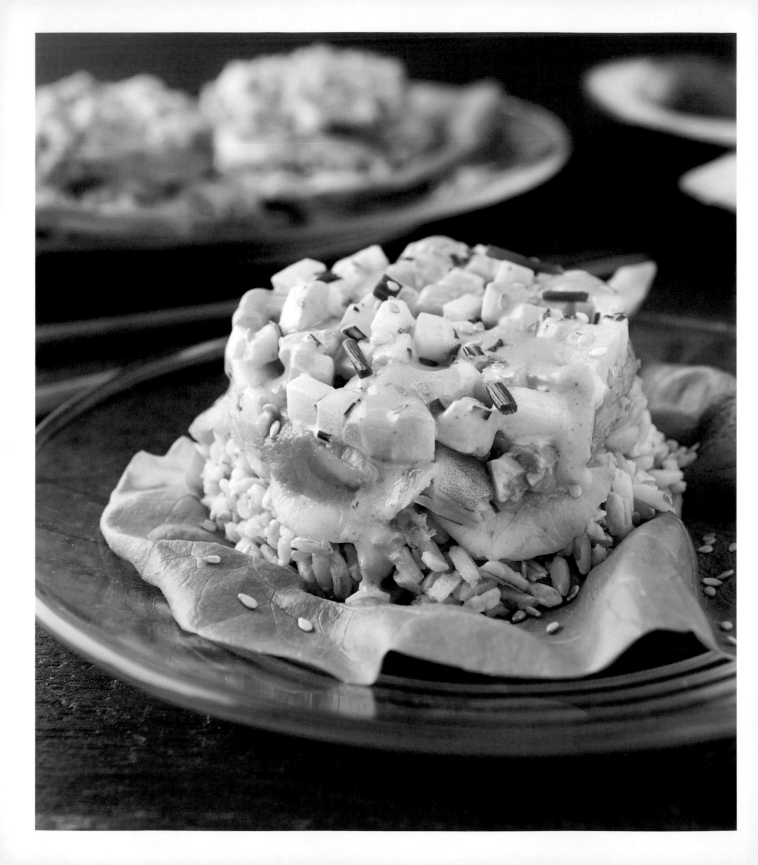

Spicy Sushi Stack

Serves 2

PUT out three small bowls. In the first, mix the rice and vinegar. In the second, toss together the cucumber, 1 tablespoon of the mayonnaise, and the chives. In the third, whisk together the remaining 1 tablespoon mayonnaise, the sesame oil, and the chile paste.

SET out two plates. Put a lettuce leaf on each plate. In a 1-cup dry measuring cup, put half the cucumber mixture, then half the avocado, half the shrimp, and half the rice. Pack it all down, then invert the cup onto one of the lettuce leaves. Carefully remove the cup so the filling stays in a cylinder shape (you may have to tap it lightly). Repeat with the remaining ingredients on the other lettuce leaf. Drizzle each stack with the chile paste mixture and sprinkle with sesame seeds and red pepper flakes.

VARIATIONS

- Serve with a side of wasabi.
- Make this with quinoa instead of brown rice.
- Use cubed sashimi-grade raw tuna instead of shrimp.

1 cup cooked short-grain brown rice, cooled but not refrigerated

1 tablespoon unseasoned rice vinegar

1 cup peeled, seeded, and cubed cucumber

2 tablespoons safflower mayonnaise

1 teaspoon chopped fresh chives

1 teaspoon toasted sesame oil

½ teaspoon red chile paste

2 large butter lettuce leaves

1 small avocado, cut into small cubes

12 ounces cooked shrimp, peeled, deveined, and cut into ½-inch pieces

4 teaspoons sesame seeds

Dashes of red pepper flakes

DINNERS

Apple-Stuffed Chicken Breasts with Kale Pesto

Serves 4

PREHEAT the oven to 375°F. Line a rimmed baking sheet with aluminum foil and put a wire rack on top.

IN a high-powered blender or food processor, pulse the garlic to coarsely chop it. Add the kale, walnuts, olive oil, lemon juice, thyme, ½ teaspoon of the salt, and ⅛ teaspoon of the pepper. Blend until smooth—this is your pesto.

SLICE each chicken breast horizontally, but not all the way through—leave it attached at one side and open it like a book. Cover with plastic wrap and pound with a kitchen mallet to about ¼ inch thick. Season both sides of the chicken with ¼ teaspoon salt and ⅛ teaspoon pepper. Spread one-quarter of the pesto over each chicken breast. Top with the apple slices. Roll up the chicken breasts with the apple slices inside and wrap 2 slices of bacon around each roll, securing it with toothpicks.

ARRANGE the chicken breasts on the rack on the prepared baking sheet. Bake for 30 minutes. Turn on the broiler and broil the chicken for 5 minutes to crisp the bacon.

TO serve, divide the romaine lettuce among four plates and top each with a chicken breast.

1 garlic clove

2 cups chopped kale

½ cup raw walnuts

2½ tablespoons olive oil

4 teaspoons fresh lemon juice

½ teaspoon fresh thyme leaves

¾ teaspoon sea salt

¼ teaspoon freshly ground black pepper

4 small boneless, skinless chicken breasts

1½ cups thinly sliced peeled apples

8 slices nitrate-free, no-sugar-added turkey bacon

8 cups chopped romaine lettuce

VARIATIONS

- Make this with turkey breasts or skirt steak instead of chicken.
- Try pears, peaches, nectarines, or plums instead of apples.

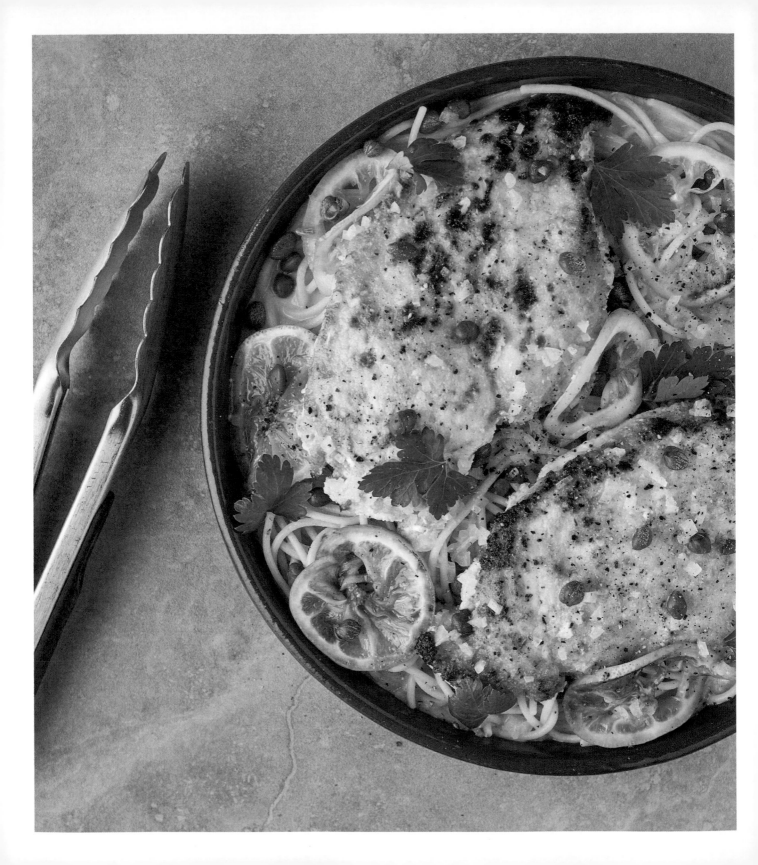

Chicken Piccata

Serves 4

PREHEAT the oven to 250°F. Place a shallow baking pan in the oven—you will use this to keep the chicken warm.

PUT the chicken breasts between two sheets of plastic wrap and pound them with a kitchen mallet until they are about ½ inch thick.

BRING a large pot of water to a boil over high heat. Add the vermicelli and cook according to the package directions. Drain and set aside.

MEANWHILE, in a large skillet, heat 2 tablespoons of the olive oil over medium-high heat. Put the flour on a shallow bowl or plate and sprinkle the salt and pepper over it. Dredge the chicken breasts in the flour mixture, shaking off any excess, and place two of them into the skillet. Cook for 4 minutes on each side, or until the chicken is cooked through, golden brown, and crispy. Transfer the chicken to the pan in the oven. Heat the remaining 2 tablespoons olive oil and repeat with the remaining two chicken breasts.

ADD the shallot to the pan and sauté, stirring continuously, for 2 minutes. Add the broth and stir, scraping up any stuck pieces from the bottom of the pan. Stir in the lemon juice, coconut milk, and capers. Bring the sauce to a low simmer and cook, stirring continuously, for 3 minutes. Remove from the heat.

TO serve, divide the vermicelli among four plates. Top each with a chicken breast. Cover each chicken breast with sauce. Garnish with the lemon slices and parsley.

4 boneless, skinless chicken breasts

12 ounces brown rice vermicelli (angel hair) pasta

4 tablespoons olive oil

¼ cup oat flour or almond flour

½ teaspoon sea salt

¼ teaspoon freshly ground black pepper

1 shallot, minced

1 cup chicken broth

Juice of 2 lemons, plus 8 thin slices lemon

½ cup coconut milk or unsweetened almond milk creamer

¼ cup capers

¼ cup chopped fresh flat-leaf parsley leaves

Muffin Tin Chicken Potpies

Serves 6

PREHEAT the oven to 350°F. Grease a muffin tin with coconut oil and set it on a baking sheet.

MAKE the gravy: In a medium saucepan, combine the cauliflower, broth, and garlic. Bring to a boil, reduce the heat to maintain a brisk simmer, and cook for 15 minutes. Stir in the paprika and salt. Carefully transfer the mixture to a blender and puree. Set aside.

MAKE the filling: In a large, heavy skillet, heat 1 tablespoon of the olive oil over medium-high heat. Add the chicken and cook, stirring occasionally, until the chicken is thoroughly browned. Season the chicken with salt and pepper and transfer to a plate.

RETURN the skillet to the heat. Add the remaining 1 tablespoon olive oil, the onions, carrots, celery, and thyme. Cook, stirring often, until the carrots and celery are soft and the onions are slightly brown on the edges, about 12 minutes.

ADD the broth and vinegar and stir, scraping up the browned bits from the bottom of the pan. Stir in the browned chicken and any accumulated juices, as well as the cauliflower puree. Remove from the heat and season with salt and pepper.

MAKE the crust: In a food processor, combine the oat flour, almond flour, salt, and eggs. Process to combine (the mixture will look like sand). Add the coconut oil and process again (the mixture should start to form clumps). Gather the dough into a ball.

Gravy

4 cups cauliflower florets, finely chopped

1½ cups chicken broth

1 garlic clove

2 teaspoons paprika

¼ teaspoon sea salt

Filling

2 tablespoons olive oil

12 ounces boneless, skinless chicken breast, diced small

Sea salt and freshly ground black pepper

3 cups diced onions

3 cups diced carrots

2 cups finely diced celery

1 teaspoon dried thyme

½ cup chicken broth

1 tablespoon white wine vinegar

Crust

2¼ cups oat flour

1½ cups almond flour

½ teaspoon sea salt

3 large eggs

3 tablespoons coconut oil

ROLL out the dough between two large sheets of parchment paper to about ⅛ inch thick. Cut circles of dough larger than the muffin cups (a Tupperware-type container or lid works well here). Press these into the muffin cups, using your fingers to press the dough into the corners and letting it rise above the rim of the cup and overlap the top of the pan a bit.

DIVIDE the filling evenly among the muffin cups. Reroll the scraps of dough and cut more circles. Top each muffin cup with a circle of dough, pressing the edges to seal the top and bottom crusts. Trim away any excess dough and use the tines of a fork to crimp the edges. Poke a couple of holes in the top crusts with the fork or a toothpick to allow steam to escape.

BAKE for 35 to 40 minutes, until browned. Let cool in the tin on a wire rack for about 5 minutes before removing the potpies from the tin and serving.

Slow Cooker Roasted Mediterranean Chicken

Serves 6

POUR the broth into a slow cooker. Add the chicken thighs, then cover them with the asparagus, mushrooms, bell peppers, onion, zucchini, cherry tomatoes, and olives. Sprinkle the oregano, basil, rosemary, salt, and pepper over the vegetables. Add the beans last. Cover and cook on low for 6 to 8 hours.

REMOVE the chicken thighs and put them in a casserole or other shallow serving dish. Spoon the contents of the slow cooker over the chicken, then drizzle with the olive oil and vinegar. Top with the parsley and serve.

1 cup chicken broth

6 boneless, skinless chicken thighs or breasts

1 pound fresh asparagus spears, cut into 2-inch pieces

8 ounces white mushrooms, sliced

1 red bell pepper, cubed

1 green bell pepper, cubed

1 red onion, sliced

1 small zucchini, quartered lengthwise, then sliced crosswise

1 cup cherry tomatoes, halved

⅓ cup pitted kalamata olives

1 tablespoon chopped fresh oregano, or 1 teaspoon dried

1 tablespoon chopped fresh basil

1 teaspoon chopped fresh rosemary

½ teaspoon sea salt

¼ teaspoon freshly ground black pepper

1 (15-ounce) can cannellini beans, drained and rinsed

2 tablespoons olive oil

2 tablespoons balsamic vinegar

2 tablespoons chopped fresh flat-leaf parsley leaves

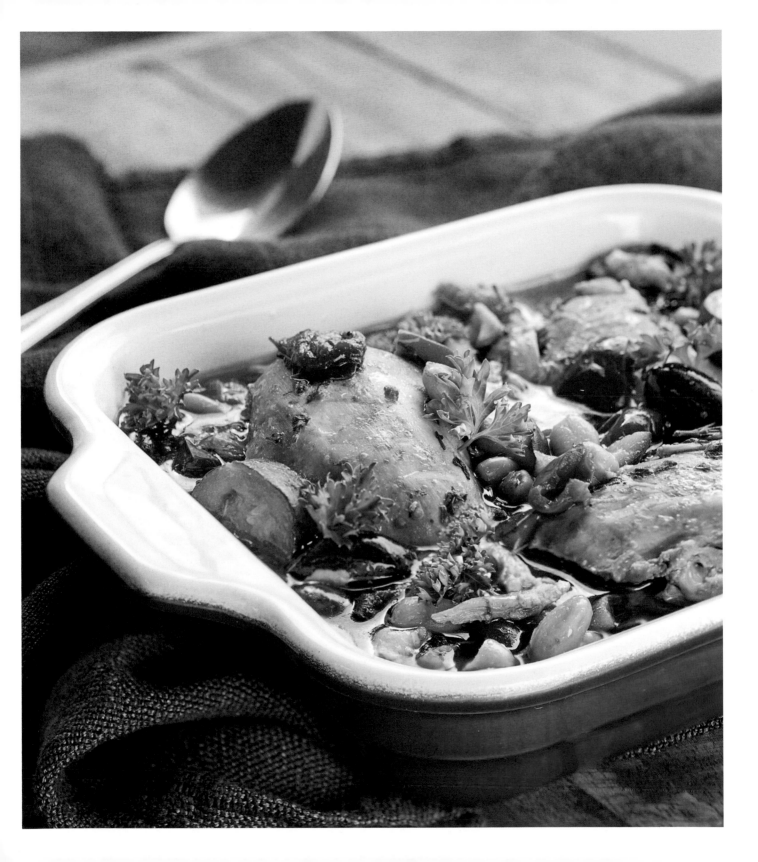

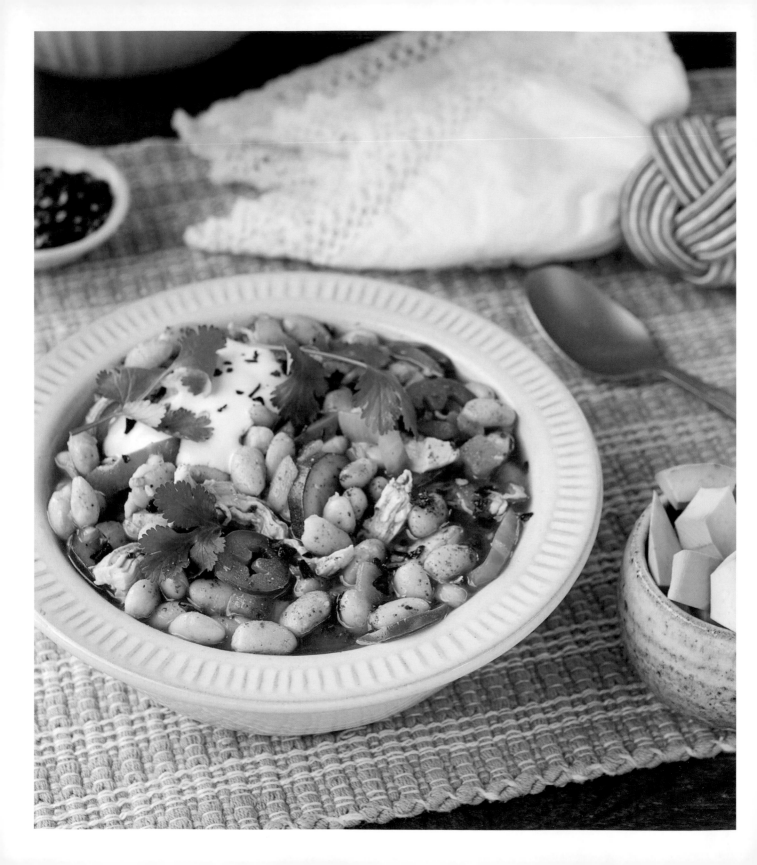

White Chicken Chili

Serves 4

IN a large soup pot or Dutch oven, heat the olive oil over medium heat. When it is hot, add the onion and sauté for 5 minutes. Add the zucchini, bell pepper, and jalapeños. Sauté for 5 minutes more. Add the green chiles, garlic, chili powder, cumin, oregano, thyme, salt, coriander, and black pepper. Sauté for 2 minutes more. Add the chicken breasts and broth. Bring the chili to a boil, then lower the heat to medium-low and cover. Simmer for 20 minutes, or until the chicken is cooked through.

REMOVE the chicken from the pot and put it on a cutting board. Using two forks, shred the meat, then return it to the pot, along with any juices from the cutting board. Add the beans. Simmer, uncovered, for 10 minutes more.

TO serve, ladle into bowls and top with the sour cream, avocado, cilantro, and red pepper flakes.

NOTE: Puree one can of the beans if you like a creamier chili.

VARIATIONS
- Make this with turkey instead of chicken.
- Make a vegetarian version by replacing the chicken with an additional can of white beans.

1 tablespoon olive oil

1 medium white onion, cut into small cubes

1 medium zucchini, cut into small cubes

1 orange (or any color) bell pepper, cut into small cubes

2 small jalapeños, seeded and minced

1 (4-ounce) can diced green chiles

3 garlic cloves, minced

1 heaping tablespoon chili powder

1 teaspoon ground cumin

1 teaspoon dried oregano

1 teaspoon dried thyme

1 teaspoon sea salt

½ teaspoon ground coriander

½ teaspoon freshly ground black pepper

4 boneless, skinless chicken breasts

4 cups chicken broth

3 (15-ounce) cans white beans, drained and rinsed (see Note)

¼ cup (4 tablespoons) Coconut Sour Cream (page 263) or Cashew Sour Cream (page 263)

1 avocado, cut into cubes

½ cup chopped fresh cilantro leaves

½ to 1 teaspoon red pepper flakes

Chicken and Black Bean Tortilla Soup

Serves 6

PREHEAT the oven to 350°F. Line a baking sheet with parchment paper.

IN a large soup pot or Dutch oven, heat the olive oil over medium heat. Add the onion and cook until soft, about 8 minutes. Add the garlic and jalapeño. Cook for 2 minutes more. Add the broth, crushed tomatoes, diced tomatoes with green chiles, chicken breasts, cumin, and chili powder. Cover and bring the soup to a simmer, then uncover and simmer for 20 minutes more.

MEANWHILE, spread out the tortilla strips on the prepared baking sheet. Bake until crisp, about 12 minutes.

REMOVE the chicken breasts and transfer them to a cutting board. Shred the meat with two forks. Stir the shredded chicken back into the soup, along with the beans and cilantro. Return the soup to a simmer and cook for 10 minutes more.

LADLE the soup into six bowls and top with the cheese (if using), tortilla strips, avocado, and sour cream (if using). Serve with the lime wedges alongside.

1 tablespoon olive oil

1 white onion, chopped

3 large garlic cloves, minced

1 jalapeño, seeded and minced

3 cups chicken broth

1 (14.5-ounce) can crushed tomatoes

1 (14.5-ounce) can diced tomatoes with green chiles

8 ounces boneless, skinless chicken breasts

1 teaspoon ground cumin

1 teaspoon chili powder

3 (8-inch) sprouted-grain tortillas, cut into thin strips

1 (14.5-ounce) can black beans, drained and rinsed

¼ cup chopped fresh cilantro

½ cup shredded almond cheese or other dairy-free, soy-free cheese (store-bought, or make your own with the recipe on page 264; optional)

1 avocado, cubed

¼ cup Coconut Sour Cream (page 263) or Cashew Sour Cream (page 263) (optional)

1 lime, cut into wedges

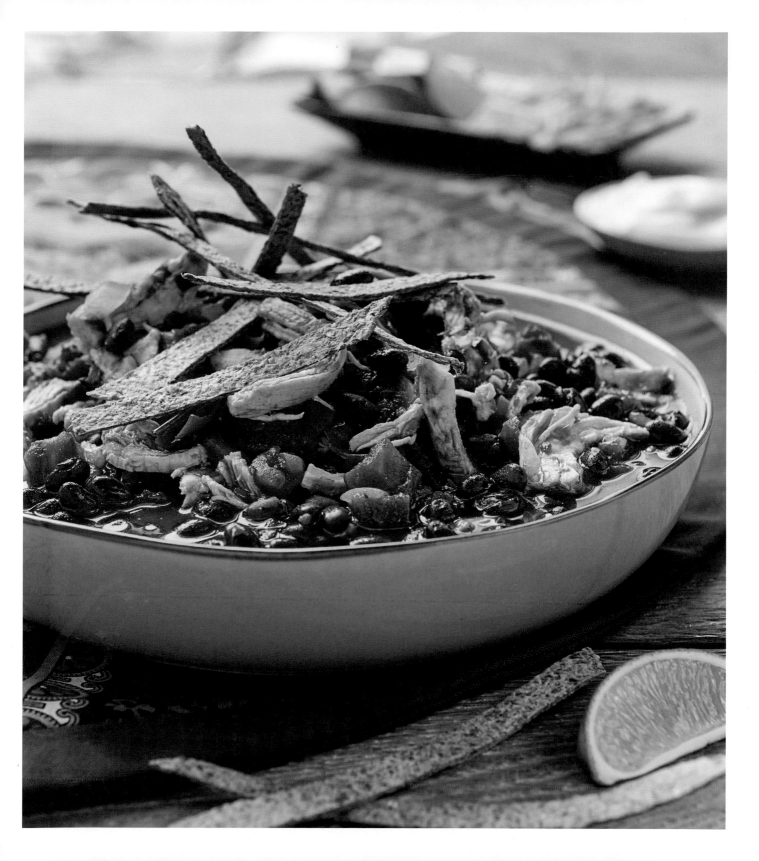

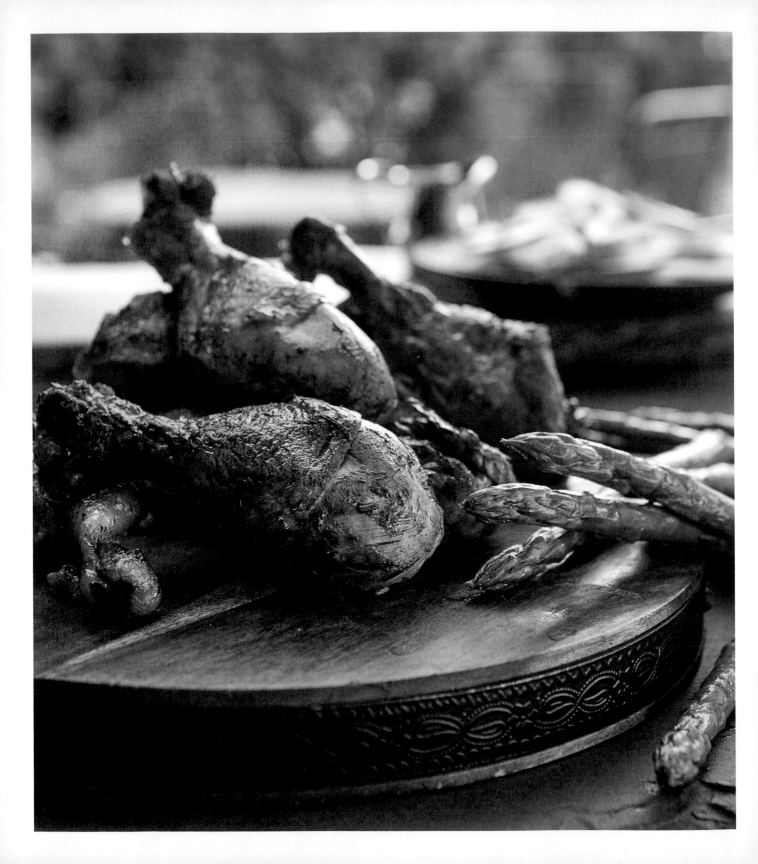

Slow Cooker Greek Drumsticks with Asparagus

Serves 4

IN a large bowl, stir together the sour cream, lemon juice, garlic, basil, oregano, parsley, dill, rosemary, marjoram, thyme, cinnamon, salt, and pepper until combined. Add the drumsticks and toss to coat all the chicken with the sauce.

PUT the drumsticks in the slow cooker. Cover and cook on high for 3 hours. Add the asparagus and cook for 1 hour more.

JUST before serving, preheat the broiler. Lightly grease a broiler pan with the grapeseed oil.

PUT the drumsticks in the prepared pan in a single layer. Broil for 6 minutes, turning the drumsticks halfway through.

DIVIDE the drumsticks among four plates. Divide the asparagus among the plates as well. Drizzle any remaining sauce and juices from the slow cooker over the asparagus and serve.

1 cup Coconut Sour Cream (page 263) or Cashew Sour Cream (page 263)

Juice of 1 lemon

2 garlic cloves, minced

4 large fresh basil leaves, minced

1 teaspoon dried oregano

1 teaspoon dried parsley

1 teaspoon chopped fresh dill

½ teaspoon dried rosemary

½ teaspoon dried marjoram

½ teaspoon dried thyme

½ teaspoon ground cinnamon

½ teaspoon sea salt

½ teaspoon freshly ground black pepper

2 pounds chicken drumsticks

2 pounds asparagus spears, trimmed and cut to fit the bottom of your slow cooker, if necessary

1 teaspoon grapeseed oil

Easy Turkey Noodle Casserole

Serves 4

PREHEAT the oven to 375°F. Line a 9-inch square (or similar size) casserole dish or baking pan with parchment paper.

IN a large deep skillet, heat the olive oil over medium-high heat. Add the turkey and onion. Sauté until the onion is soft, about 5 minutes. Add the celery, carrots, zucchini, green beans, and garlic. Sauté for 8 minutes, or until all the vegetables are tender. Stir in the arrowroot mixture, almond milk, salt, and pepper. Lower the heat to medium-low, cover, and simmer the sauce for 10 minutes.

MEANWHILE, cook the penne according to the package directions.

UNCOVER the sauce and remove it from the heat. Drain the pasta but don't rinse it. Stir the hot pasta into the sauce, then add the parsley and stir to combine everything. Transfer the mixture to the prepared casserole dish. Sprinkle with the paprika. Bake the casserole for 30 minutes, or until bubbling and just starting to brown on top. Remove from the oven and let cool for 10 minutes before scooping the casserole into bowls and serving.

1 tablespoon olive oil

8 ounces turkey breast, cut into 1-inch pieces

1 medium yellow onion, chopped

4 celery stalks, thinly sliced

2 medium carrots, halved lengthwise and sliced

1 small zucchini, halved lengthwise and sliced

1 cup chopped green beans (chop into ½-inch pieces)

4 garlic cloves, minced

1 tablespoon arrowroot powder, mixed with 1 tablespoon water

2 cups unsweetened almond milk

2 teaspoons sea salt

½ teaspoon freshly ground black pepper

8 ounces brown rice penne

¼ cup minced fresh flat-leaf parsley leaves

½ teaspoon smoked paprika

VARIATIONS

- Use chicken instead of turkey.
- Use 1 (15-ounce) can white beans or chickpeas, drained and rinsed, instead of turkey for a vegetarian version.
- Use any other shape or type of pasta, as long as it is wheat-free and corn-free.
- Use brown rice instead of pasta.

Sweet-and-Sour Chicken

Serves 4

IN a small bowl, combine the coconut aminos, vinegar, ketchup, garlic, five-spice powder, and salt. Set aside.

IN a large skillet, heat the sesame oil over medium-high heat. Add the chicken and cook, without stirring, for 2 minutes. Flip the chicken pieces over and cook for 2 minutes more. Stir in the onion, bell peppers, and pineapple chunks. Cook for 3 minutes.

STIR in the sauce and the pineapple puree. Add ¼ cup warm water and bring to a simmer. Reduce the heat to medium. Cook, stirring occasionally, for 10 to 15 minutes, until the chicken is cooked through.

REMOVE the chicken and vegetables with a slotted spoon and put them on a plate, leaving just the liquid in the skillet. Stir the arrowroot mixture into the skillet. Bring to a simmer and cook, stirring often, until the mixture thickens, about 5 minutes. Return the chicken and veggies to the skillet and stir to coat with the sauce.

TO serve, divide the cauliflower rice among four plates. Top with the chicken. Garnish each serving with cilantro, scallions, and sesame seeds.

NOTE: Buy cauliflower rice fresh or frozen from the supermarket, or coarsely chop fresh cauliflower florets in a food processor until they're broken down into pieces the size of rice.

½ cup coconut aminos

⅓ cup unseasoned rice vinegar

⅓ cup no-sugar-added ketchup

1 tablespoon minced garlic

1 teaspoon Chinese five-spice powder

½ teaspoon sea salt

2 tablespoons sesame oil

1 pound boneless, skinless chicken breast, cut into 1½- to 2-inch pieces

1 medium red onion, cut into 1-inch pieces

2 red bell peppers, cut into 1- to 2-inch pieces

1 yellow bell pepper, cut into 1- to 2-inch pieces

¾ cup fresh pineapple chunks

⅔ cup pureed fresh pineapple

2 tablespoons arrowroot powder, mixed with ⅓ cup cold water

4 cups cooked cauliflower rice (see Note), for serving

¼ cup chopped fresh cilantro

2 scallions, thinly sliced

4 teaspoons sesame seeds

VARIATION

- You could serve this over brown rice or quinoa instead of the cauliflower rice.

Jerk Turkey Kebabs with Creamy Jicama Slaw

Serves 4

PREHEAT a grill to 400°F or preheat the broiler.

IN a shallow bowl or large zip-top bag, combine the thyme, garlic powder, allspice, salt, ¼ teaspoon of the cinnamon, the black pepper, ginger, nutmeg, and cayenne. Add the turkey and mix to coat all the pieces with the seasoning. Set aside. Put the pineapple chunks in a small bowl and sprinkle with the paprika and remaining ¼ teaspoon cinnamon. Using metal skewers or wooden skewers soaked in water for 15 minutes, thread one piece each of the turkey, pineapple chunks, bell peppers of each color, onions, and mushrooms onto a skewer, then repeat until the skewer is full. Fill the other skewers.

GRILL the kebabs for 25 minutes, turning them every 5 minutes to cook evenly. If broiling, broil for 8 minutes, turning the kebabs every 2 minutes.

SERVE with creamy slaw alongside.

2 teaspoons dried thyme

1 teaspoon garlic powder

½ teaspoon ground allspice

½ teaspoon sea salt

½ teaspoon ground cinnamon

¼ teaspoon freshly ground black pepper

¼ teaspoon ground ginger

¼ teaspoon ground nutmeg

¼ teaspoon cayenne pepper

1 pound boneless, skinless turkey breast, cut into bite-size cubes

1 large pineapple, cubed, or 1 (20-ounce) can pineapple chunks in juice, drained

1 teaspoon smoked paprika

1 large red bell pepper, cut into bite-size chunks

1 large yellow bell pepper, cut into bite-size chunks

2 large red onions, cut into bite-size chunks

8 ounces white, cremini, or baby bella mushrooms, stems trimmed but left attached

Creamy Jicama Slaw (page 200)

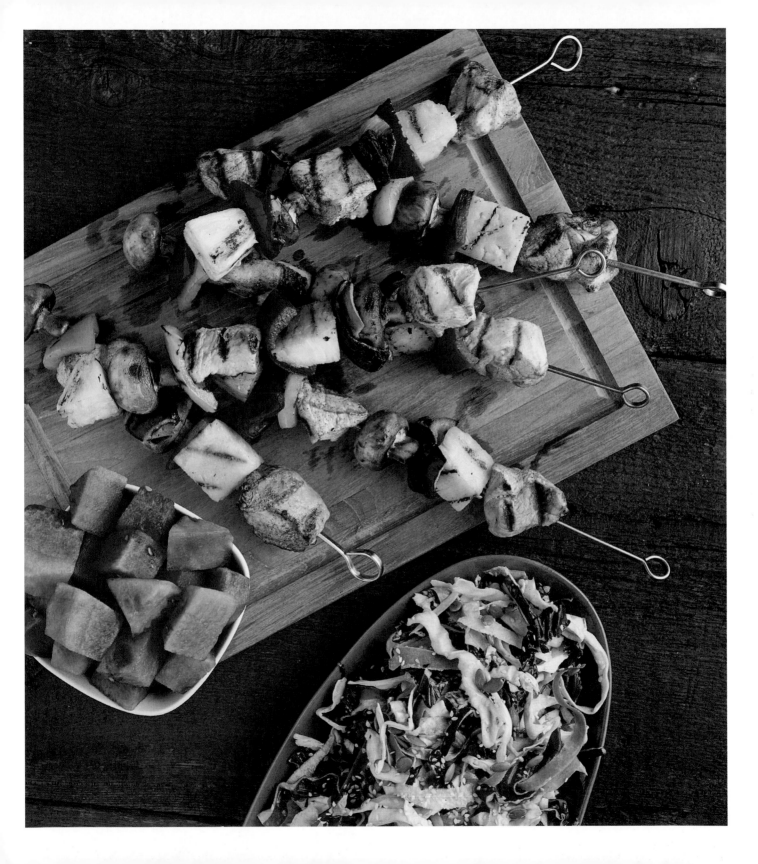

Creamy Jicama Slaw

Serves 4

IN a large bowl, combine all the ingredients and mix until everything is fully combined.

1 cup shredded jicama

1 cup shredded green cabbage

1 cup shredded purple cabbage

1 cup shredded carrots

½ cup shredded radishes

½ cup safflower mayonnaise or avocado mayonnaise

¼ cup raw pumpkin seeds (pepitas)

¼ cup raw sesame seeds

¼ cup chopped fresh cilantro leaves

Juice of ½ lemon

½ teaspoon smoked paprika

½ teaspoon sea salt

½ teaspoon freshly ground black pepper

VARIATIONS

- Use chicken or steak cubes instead of turkey.
- Use other vegetables on the kebabs, such as zucchini cubes or cherry tomatoes.
- Use other fruit, such as peaches or watermelon.
- Leave the jicama out of the coleslaw and increase the cabbage by 1 cup.

Loaded Cowboy Burgers

Serves 4

PREHEAT the oven to 400°F. Line a rimmed baking sheet with parchment paper.

IN a large bowl, combine the ground beef, carrot, bacon, spinach, red onion, egg whites, cilantro, 1 tablespoon of the coconut aminos, the mustard, jalapeño, garlic, salt, pepper and sriracha (if using). Mix with your hands to combine everything thoroughly. Add the oats and mix again until they are fully incorporated. Form the beef mixture into four patties. Put them on the prepared baking sheet and bake for 20 minutes (or to your desired doneness), carefully flipping the burgers halfway through. During the last 8 minutes of cooking, open the buns and put them in the oven, directly on an oven rack, to toast.

MEANWHILE, in a large skillet, heat the broth over medium-high heat. Add the sweet onion, mushrooms, remaining 1 table-spoon coconut aminos, and the vinegar. Sauté until the onion is very soft and dark, the mushrooms have shrunk down, and all the liquid has evaporated (you may need to add more broth while cooking). Remove from the heat.

ON the bottom half of each bun, put a burger and top with one-quarter of the onion-mushroom mixture. Add any other top-pings you like. Cover with the top of the bun and serve.

VARIATIONS

- You could make this recipe with ground turkey.
- Pair this burger with oven-baked sweet potato fries (see page 165).

1 pound extra-lean ground beef

1 medium carrot, grated

4 slices nitrate-free, no-sugar-added turkey bacon, cooked and crumbled

½ cup frozen chopped spinach, defrosted and drained

½ small red onion, finely chopped

2 egg whites

2 tablespoons finely chopped fresh cilantro

2 tablespoons coconut aminos

1 tablespoon Dijon mustard (no sugar added)

1 jalapeño, seeded and minced

1 garlic clove, minced

½ teaspoon sea salt

¼ teaspoon freshly ground black pepper

A few dashes of sriracha or your favorite hot sauce (optional)

¼ cup quick-cooking oats

4 sprouted-grain buns

½ cup beef broth or vegetable broth, or a little more if needed

1 cup thinly sliced sweet onion

8 ounces white mushrooms, sliced

1 tablespoon balsamic vinegar

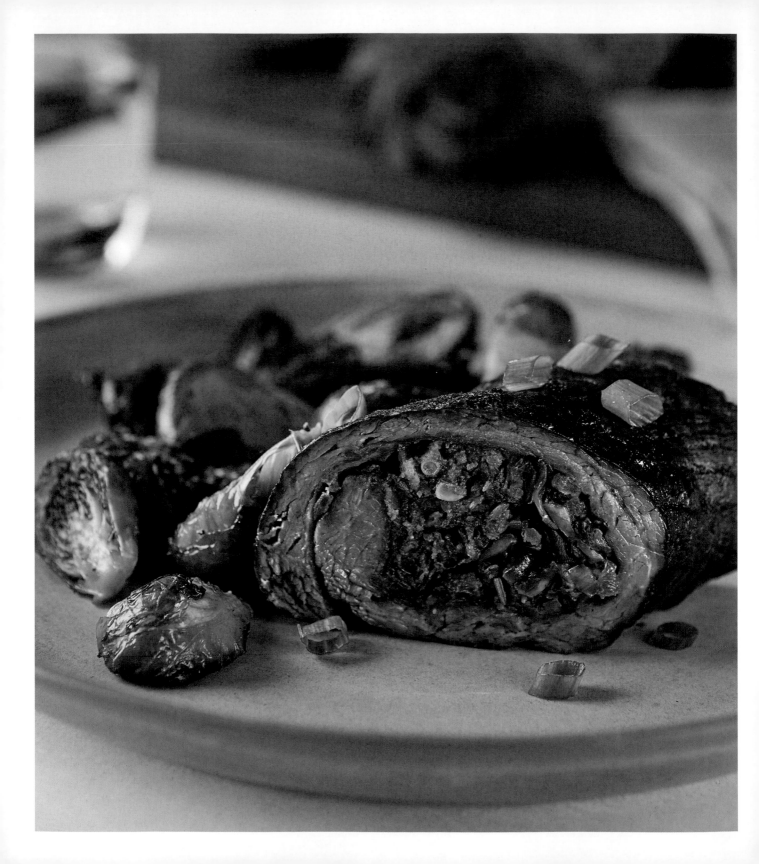

Spinach-and-Mushroom-Stuffed Flank Steak

Serves 4

PREHEAT the oven to 350°F. Line two baking sheets with parchment paper.

IN a medium skillet, heat 1 tablespoon of the olive oil over medium-high heat. Add the mushrooms and onion and sauté until the onion is just turning golden brown, about 8 minutes. Add the garlic and sauté for 2 minutes more. Stir in the rosemary, liquid aminos, ½ teaspoon of the salt, and ½ teaspoon of the pepper. Remove from the heat and set aside.

ON a large cutting board, lay out the steaks. Cover each one with one-quarter of the mushroom mixture, spreading it almost to the edges. Top each with one-quarter of the bread crumbs and ¼ cup of the spinach and drizzle with 1 tablespoon of the olive oil. Tightly roll up the steaks, securing them with toothpicks, and put them on one of the prepared baking sheets.

IN a large bowl, toss the Brussels sprouts with the remaining 1 tablespoon olive oil and remaining ½ teaspoon each salt and pepper. Spread them out on the other baking sheet.

PUT both baking sheets in the oven, steak on top, Brussels sprouts below, and bake for 30 minutes. Remove the steak from the oven and cover with aluminum foil. Turn on the broiler and move the Brussels sprouts to the top rack. Broil the Brussels sprouts for about 5 minutes, or until they start to look crispy (they can burn fast, so watch them closely). Remove them from the oven.

UNCOVER the steak rolls and slice each in half crosswise. Separate the halves and arrange them in a V shape on a plate. Drizzle with any juices left in the pan and top with the scallions. Serve with the Brussels sprouts on the side.

3 tablespoons olive oil

1½ cups finely chopped white mushrooms

½ cup finely chopped yellow onion

2 garlic cloves, minced

1 teaspoon fresh rosemary

1 tablespoon liquid aminos

1 teaspoon sea salt

1 teaspoon freshly ground black pepper

1 pound flank steak, cut into 4 pieces, each piece butterflied

1 slice sprouted-grain bread, toasted and chopped into crumbs

1 cup fresh baby spinach

1 pound fresh Brussels sprouts, trimmed and cut in half

6 tablespoons thinly sliced scallions

Mongolian Beef over Cauliflower Rice

Serves 6

IN a large bowl or zip-top plastic bag, toss the sliced steak with the arrowroot.

IN the bottom of a slow cooker, combine the grapeseed oil, garlic, ginger, water, tamari, xylitol, and chile paste. Add the steak, carrots, bell peppers, and ¾ cup of the scallions. Stir to coat everything.

COVER and cook on high for 3 to 4 hours or on low for 6 hours, until the steak is cooked through and tender.

WHEN ready to serve, heat a large skillet over medium-high heat, add a tablespoon or two of oil (or broth), and sauté the cauliflower rice for 3 to 4 minutes, until tender.

SERVE the beef mixture over the cooked cauliflower rice, sprinkled with the remaining scallions and the sesame seeds.

1½ pounds flank steak, thinly sliced (¼ inch thick)

3 tablespoons arrowroot powder

1 tablespoon grapeseed oil, plus more for the cauliflower rice

3 or 4 garlic cloves, minced

2 teaspoons minced fresh ginger

⅓ cup water

⅓ cup tamari

⅓ cup xylitol

1 to 2 teaspoons red chile paste

2 cups shredded carrots

2 cups red bell pepper strips

¾ cup plus ½ cup sliced scallions (sliced on an angle into 1-inch pieces)

8 cups cauliflower rice (see Note, page 197)

2 tablespoons sesame seeds

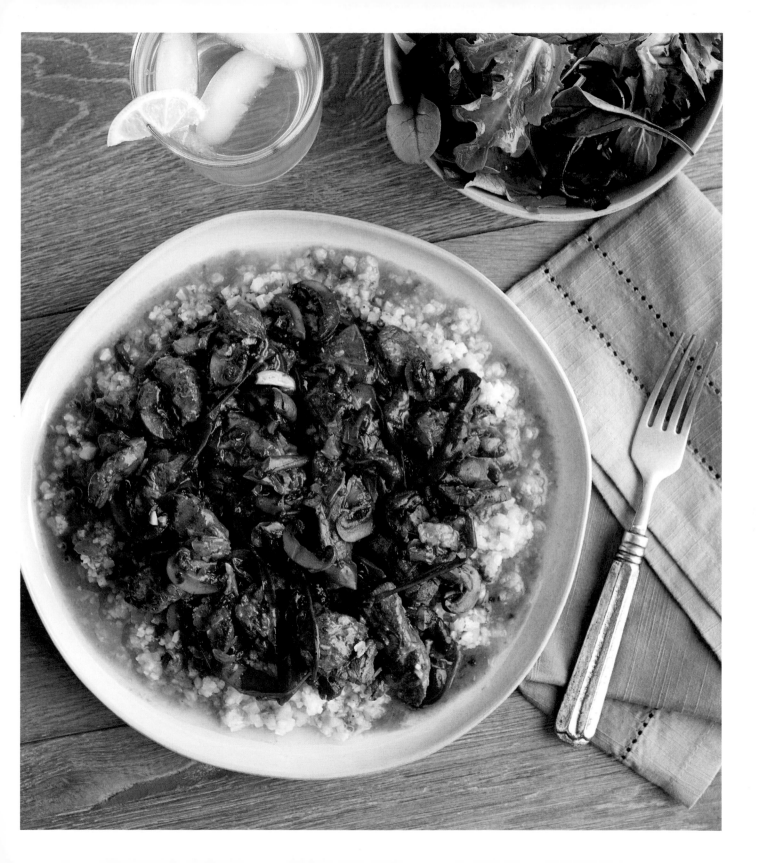

Slow Cooker Creamy Beef Stroganoff

Serves 6

PLACE the steak in a slow cooker. Cover it with the mushrooms, bell peppers, onion, and garlic.

IN a medium bowl, whisk together the arrowroot mixture, broth, tamari, vinegar, black pepper, salt, cloves, and cayenne, and pour the mixture into the slow cooker over the meat and vegetables. Cover and cook on low for 6 to 8 hours. Before serving, stir in the milk.

DIVIDE the cauliflower rice among six bowls and ladle the stroganoff over the rice. Top with the parsley and serve.

VARIATION

• Serve over brown rice fettuccine.

1½ pounds sirloin steak, thinly sliced

12 ounces cremini or baby bella mushrooms, sliced

2 red bell peppers, cut into thin strips

1 medium white onion, chopped

4 garlic cloves, minced

3 tablespoons arrowroot powder, mixed with 2 tablespoons water

1½ cups beef broth

¼ cup tamari

¼ cup red wine vinegar

1½ teaspoons freshly ground black pepper

1 teaspoon sea salt

Pinch of ground cloves

Pinch of cayenne pepper

½ cup canned coconut milk or cashew milk

6 cups cooked cauliflower rice (see Note, page 197) or long-grain brown rice

¼ cup chopped fresh flat-leaf parsley

Taco Pasta Casserole

Serves 8

PREHEAT the oven to 350°F. Line a 9×13-inch baking pan with parchment paper.

IN a large skillet, crumble the ground beef and add the onion. Sauté over medium-high until the beef is browned and the onion is soft, about 8 minutes. Add the bell peppers and jalapeño. Sauté until the bell peppers are soft, about 5 minutes more. Stir in the tomatoes, black beans, salsa, broth, ⅓ cup of the nutritional yeast, the chili powder, oregano, chipotle powder, garlic powder, onion powder, cumin, salt, and black pepper. Bring the mixture to a simmer and cook, stirring occasionally, for 10 minutes. Remove the skillet from the heat and stir in the cooked pasta. Transfer the mixture to the prepared casserole dish. Bake until bubbling, about 25 minutes.

MEANWHILE, in a medium bowl, whisk together the sour cream, lime juice, and the remaining 1 tablespoon nutritional yeast.

WHEN the casserole is done, take it out of the oven and drizzle with the sour cream mixture. Sprinkle the cilantro over the top. Scoop out portions and serve.

VARIATIONS

- Make this with ground turkey or nitrate-free, no-sugar-added turkey sausage.
- Eliminate the meat and double the black beans for a meatless version.

---

2 pounds lean ground beef

1 large white onion, finely chopped

1 green bell pepper, cut into small cubes

1 red bell pepper, cut into small cubes

1 jalapeño, seeded and minced

2 (15-ounce) cans fire-roasted diced tomatoes

1 (15-ounce) can black beans, drained and rinsed

1 cup red salsa

1 cup chicken broth or vegetable broth

⅓ cup plus 1 tablespoon nutritional yeast

1 tablespoon chili powder

2 teaspoons dried Mexican oregano

1 teaspoon chipotle powder

1 teaspoon garlic powder

1 teaspoon onion powder

½ teaspoon ground cumin

½ teaspoon sea salt

½ teaspoon freshly ground black pepper

4 cups cooked brown rice penne pasta

Coconut Sour Cream (page 263) or Cashew Sour Cream (page 263)

2 tablespoons fresh lime juice

½ cup chopped fresh cilantro leaves

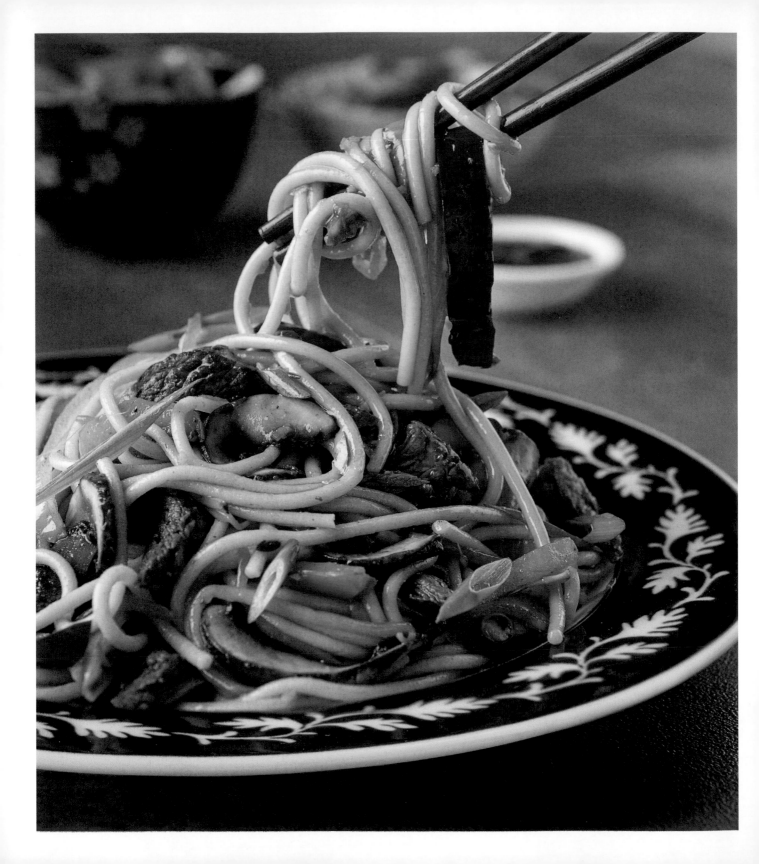

Beef Lo Mein

Serves 2

MAKE the sauce: In a small bowl, whisk together all the sauce ingredients until smooth. Set aside.

MAKE the lo mein: Cook the vermicelli according to the package directions.

IN a large nonstick skillet, sauté the beef over medium-high heat for 2 minutes, or until cooked to your preference. Transfer the beef to a plate.

IN the same skillet, combine the bell peppers, bean sprouts, curry powder, and the broth (add more, if you need it, to prevent sticking). Stir-fry for 3 minutes. Add the mushrooms and peas. Stir-fry for 2 minutes more, or until the vegetables are brightly colored and tender-crisp. Stir in the sauce and return the beef to the skillet, along with any juices. Stir and simmer until the sauce thickens, about 8 minutes. Sprinkle with the scallions and serve.

Sauce

1 cup chicken broth

¼ cup tamari

2 teaspoons minced garlic

2 teaspoons minced fresh ginger

1 teaspoon arrowroot powder

½ teaspoon red chile paste (more or less, depending on how spicy you like it)

Lo Mein

4 ounces uncooked brown rice vermicelli (angel hair)

8 ounces beef, thinly sliced

2 bell peppers (any color), thinly sliced

2 cups bean sprouts

1 teaspoon curry powder

2 tablespoons chicken broth, plus more if needed

1 cup sliced shiitake mushrooms

1 cup sugar snap peas, sliced into strips

½ cup sliced scallions

Spaghetti Bolognese

Serves 4

IN a large saucepan, heat the olive oil over medium heat. Add the ground beef, onion, and bell pepper. Sauté until the vegetables are soft, about 7 minutes. Add the mushrooms and sauté until the mushrooms shrink down, about 5 minutes. Add the garlic and sauté for 2 minutes more. Stir in the broth, diced tomatoes, tomato sauce, tomato paste, oregano, basil, salt, thyme, and pepper. Bring to a simmer, then lower the heat to medium-low and simmer for 30 minutes.

MEANWHILE, cook the spaghetti according to the package directions. Drain and rinse the spaghetti, then divide it among four plates. Top each plate with one-quarter of the sauce. Top with nutritional yeast, if desired, and serve.

VARIATIONS

- Make this with ground turkey or nitrate-free, no-sugar-added ground turkey sausage instead of ground beef.
- If you like a sweeter sauce, add 1 small grated carrot and/or 2 teaspoons xylitol to the sauce when you add the broth and tomatoes.

1 tablespoon olive oil

1 pound extra-lean ground beef

1 yellow onion, chopped

1 green bell pepper, finely chopped

1 pound white mushrooms, thinly sliced

3 garlic cloves, minced

2 cups beef broth or vegetable broth

1 (15-ounce) can fire-roasted diced tomatoes

1 (8-ounce) can tomato sauce

1 (4-ounce) can tomato paste

2 teaspoons dried oregano

1 teaspoon dried basil

1 teaspoon sea salt

½ teaspoon dried thyme

¼ teaspoon freshly ground black pepper

8 ounces brown rice spaghetti (or other wheat-free, corn-free pasta)

Nutritional yeast, for serving (optional)

Spicy Lamb Tagine

Serves 8

IN a large skillet with a lid, sauté the lamb and onions over medium heat until the lamb is browned and the onions are soft, about 5 minutes. Add the bell pepper and sauté until it is soft, about 3 minutes. Add the garlic and ginger. Sauté for 2 minutes more. Add the turmeric, cumin, coriander, paprika, harissa, salt, cinnamon, black pepper, and cardamom. Stir to coat the vegetables with the spices. Add the broth, crushed tomatoes, and tomato paste. Stir to combine everything and bring the mixture to a low boil. Reduce the heat to medium-low, cover the skillet, and cook for 30 minutes. Remove the lid and raise the heat to medium-high. Cook, stirring frequently to prevent sticking, until the tagine is thick like stew, about 10 minutes.

DIVIDE the quinoa among eight bowls and spoon the tagine over the top. Sprinkle each bowl with 1 tablespoon each of the olives, almonds, and cilantro.

VARIATIONS

- Make this with ground beef or shredded chicken breast instead of lamb.
- Make this with two sweet potatoes, peeled and diced, instead of the meat for a vegetarian version.
- Instead of olives, you could top this with chopped fresh, pitted apricots.

2 pounds ground lamb

2 yellow onions, thinly sliced

1 yellow bell pepper, cut into strips

4 garlic cloves, minced

1 (1-inch) piece fresh ginger, peeled and minced

1 tablespoon ground turmeric

1 tablespoon ground cumin

1 tablespoon ground coriander

1 tablespoon paprika

1 tablespoon harissa or red chile paste

1 teaspoon sea salt

½ teaspoon ground cinnamon

¼ teaspoon freshly ground black pepper

¼ teaspoon ground cardamom

4 cups vegetable broth

1 (28-ounce) can crushed tomatoes

¼ cup tomato paste

4 cups cooked white quinoa

½ cup pitted kalamata olives

½ cup slivered raw almonds

½ cup chopped fresh cilantro leaves

Slow Cooker Hungarian Goulash

Serves 8

PUT the beef in a slow cooker. Add the mushrooms, carrots, onion, rutabaga, parsnip, and garlic.

IN a large bowl, whisk together the tomato paste, liquid aminos, paprika, xylitol (if using), salt, and pepper. Whisk in the broth. Pour the liquid into the slow cooker over the vegetables and meat. Cover and cook on high for 6 hours. Serve topped with the parsley.

2 pounds beef stew meat

1 pound white mushrooms, sliced

4 carrots, sliced on an angle

1 large yellow onion, diced

1 rutabaga, peeled and diced

1 parsnip, peeled and sliced on an angle

3 garlic cloves, minced

¼ cup tomato paste

¼ cup liquid aminos

3 tablespoons Hungarian paprika

3 tablespoons xylitol (optional)

2 teaspoons sea salt

1 teaspoon freshly ground black pepper

4 cups beef broth

½ cup chopped fresh parsley

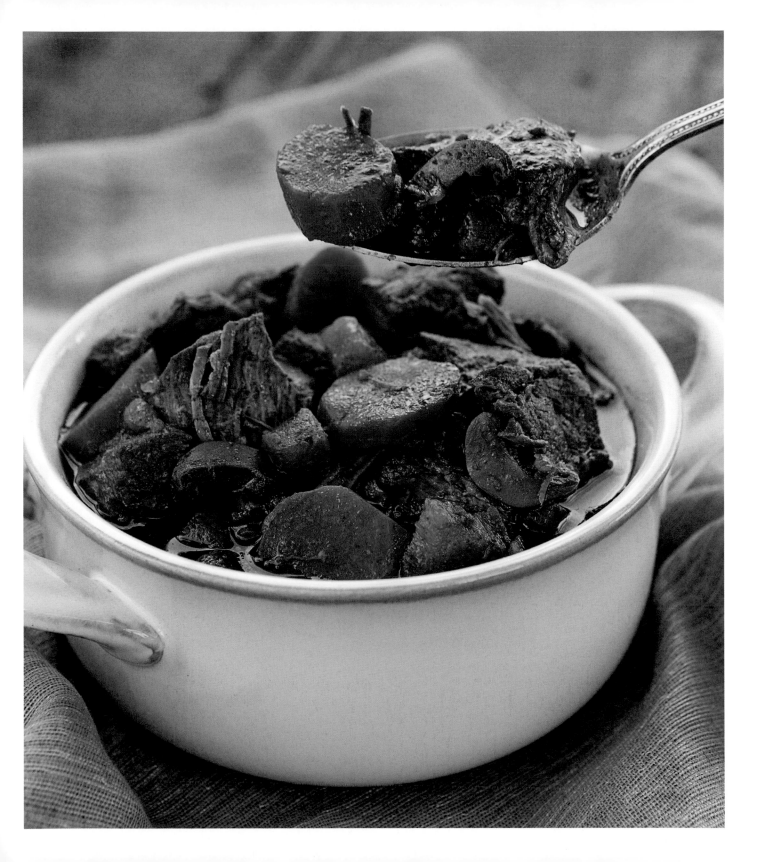

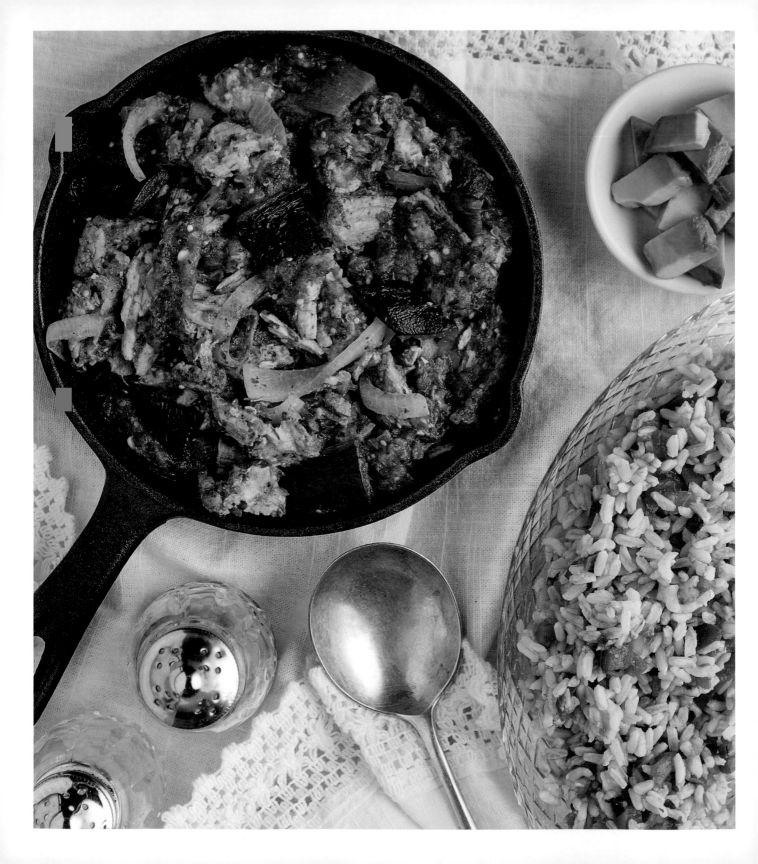

Poblano Pork Chili Verde in the Skillet

Serves 4

PREHEAT the broiler. Line a rimmed baking sheet with parchment paper.

PUT the tomatillos and peppers on the prepared baking sheet, cut-sides up, and add the garlic. Broil until all the vegetables are very soft and charred, about 12 minutes, turning the tomatillos every 2 minutes. Remove the baking sheet from the oven. Put the peppers in a paper bag and roll it shut (this will help steam off the skins). When the peppers are cool enough to handle, peel off the skins (running them under cold water can make this easier—if you can't get it all off, that's okay). Transfer half the peppers and half the tomatillos, plus any juices from the pan, to a blender. Add half the onion. Squeeze the garlic cloves out of their skins into the blender. Add the lime juice, cilantro, and salt. Blend until smooth. Coarsely chop the remaining peppers, tomatillos, and onion, keeping the onion separate.

IN a large skillet, heat the olive oil over medium heat. Add the pork loin, remaining onion, oregano, cumin, and chipotle powder. Sauté until the onion is soft and the pork loin is cooked through and lightly browned. Pour the blended pepper-tomatillo mixture, the chopped peppers and tomatillos, and the broth over the pork and mix to combine. Bring the mixture to a simmer, then reduce the heat to medium-low. Cover and cook, stirring frequently, for 20 minutes.

DIVIDE the rice among four bowls. Top each bowl with 1 tablespoon of the red salsa and mix it with the rice. Divide the pork mixture among the bowls, ladling it over the rice. Garnish with the avocado cubes and serve.

8 tomatillos, husked and rinsed well

4 poblano peppers, halved and seeded

3 Anaheim peppers or Hatch green chiles, halved and seeded

3 jalapeños, halved and seeded

2 garlic cloves, unpeeled

1 small white onion, halved

½ cup fresh lime juice

¼ cup chopped fresh cilantro leaves

½ teaspoon sea salt

1 tablespoon olive oil

1 pound pork loin, cut into chunks

2 teaspoons dried Mexican (or regular) oregano

1 teaspoon ground cumin

½ teaspoon chipotle powder

1 cup chicken broth

2 cups cooked long-grain brown rice

4 tablespoons red salsa

1 avocado, cubed

Oven-Baked Stuffed Pork Roast

Serves 8

PREHEAT the oven to 350°F. Line a roasting pan with parchment paper.

IN a large skillet, heat the olive oil over medium-high heat. Add the chopped onion and sauté until soft, about 8 minutes. Stir in the apple, squash, rice, chopped cranberries, rosemary leaves, 1 teaspoon of the salt, the thyme, ½ teaspoon of the pepper, and the cloves. Cook, stirring frequently, for 5 minutes, then remove from the heat.

CUT the pork loin into 1-inch slices but not all the way through (cut down to about 1 or 2 inches from the bottom of the roast). Put the pork in the prepared pan. Stuff the apple-squash mixture in between the slices of the roast. Season with the remaining 1 teaspoon salt and ½ teaspoon pepper. Arrange the sliced onion, whole cranberries, and rosemary sprigs around the roast. Drizzle the broth around the roast (not on top of it). Cover the pan with aluminum foil. Roast for 45 minutes, or until the internal temperature is 150 degrees, removing the foil for the last 15 minutes to brown the roast. When the roast is done, remove it from the oven, cover it with foil or a tea towel, and let it rest for 10 minutes before slicing.

SERVE with a green salad.

2 tablespoons olive oil

1 large sweet onion, halved: half finely chopped, the other half sliced

1 large apple, cored and cut into small cubes

1 cup cooked or thawed frozen butternut squash cubes

1 cup cooked wild rice

1 cup fresh or thawed frozen cranberries: half chopped and half left whole

1 tablespoon fresh rosemary leaves, plus 2 sprigs

2 teaspoons sea salt

1 teaspoon dried thyme

1 teaspoon freshly ground black pepper

¼ teaspoon ground cloves

1 (2-pound) pork loin roast

½ teaspoon freshly ground black pepper

2 cups chicken broth

Green salad, for serving

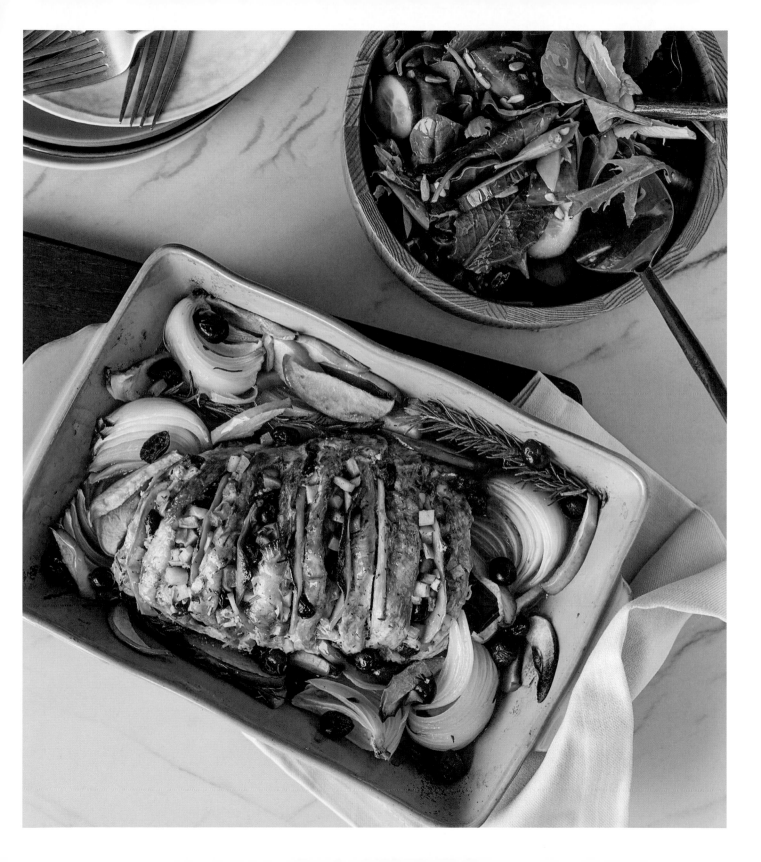

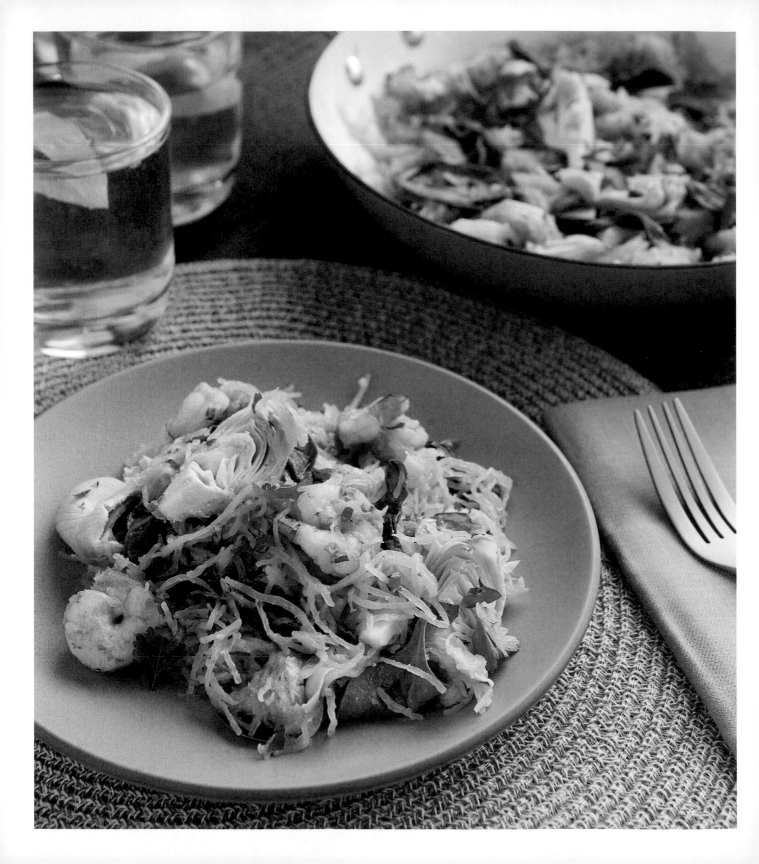

Spaghetti Squash Shrimp and Artichoke Alfredo

Serves 4

1 medium spaghetti squash

3 tablespoons olive oil

2 teaspoons sea salt

1 teaspoon freshly ground black pepper

1½ pounds raw shrimp, peeled and deveined

1 sweet onion, chopped

3 garlic cloves, minced

1 tablespoon fresh lemon juice

1 tablespoon nutritional yeast

1 teaspoon garlic powder

½ teaspoon dried oregano

1 (14-ounce) can coconut milk (not low-fat)

1 (14-ounce) can water-packed artichoke hearts, drained and cut into quarters

½ cup chicken broth

1 cup baby spinach

¼ cup chopped fresh parsley leaves

PREHEAT the oven to 400°F. Line a baking pan with parchment paper.

CUT the spaghetti squash in half lengthwise. Scoop out the seeds. Drizzle with 2 teaspoons olive oil and sprinkle with salt and pepper. Put the squash halves cut-side down in the pan. Roast for 1 hour. Remove from the oven and set aside to cool.

IN a large skillet, heat 1 tablespoon olive oil over medium-high heat. Add the shrimp and sauté, stirring continuously, until the shrimp turn pink, about 4 minutes. Transfer the shrimp to a plate and set aside. Add the remaining olive oil to the pan. Add the onion and sauté until soft, about 5 minutes. Add the garlic and sauté for 2 minutes more. Add the lemon juice, nutritional yeast, garlic powder, and oregano and sauté for 1 minute. Stir in the coconut milk, artichoke hearts, and broth. Lower the heat to medium-low. Simmer, stirring frequently, for 20 minutes. Remove from the heat and stir in the spinach.

MEANWHILE, using a fork, scrape the flesh of the spaghetti squash from the shells to form "noodles" and divide them among four plates.

TOP the squash noodles with the sauce, garnish with the parsley, and serve.

VARIATIONS

- Serve over brown rice linguine (or any other wheat-free, corn-free pasta).
- Use chicken cut into bite-size pieces instead of shrimp.

Spicy Caribbean Shrimp Curry

Serves 4

IN a medium bowl, whisk together the turmeric, cumin, thyme, coriander, allspice, ginger, mustard, fenugreek, black pepper, cloves, nutmeg, and cayenne. Add the shrimp and toss to coat with the spices. Set aside.

IN a large skillet, heat the safflower oil over medium-high heat. Add the onion and sauté until soft, about 5 minutes. Add the bell peppers, zucchini, and carrot. Sauté until the vegetables are soft, about 5 minutes. Add the garlic and sauté for 2 minutes more. Scoop the shrimp out of the spice mixture and set them aside on a plate. Add the spice mixture to the skillet and sauté for 2 minutes, stirring to cover the vegetables in the spices. Stir in the broth and tomatoes. Bring the sauce to a simmer, then lower the heat to medium-low and simmer until the sauce thickens, about 10 minutes. Stir in the shrimp and cook until the shrimp turn pink, about 5 minutes more.

DIVIDE the rice among four bowls. Ladle the curry over the rice. Garnish with the scallions and serve.

- 1 tablespoon ground turmeric
- 2 teaspoons ground cumin
- 1 teaspoon fresh thyme, or ½ teaspoon dried
- ½ teaspoon ground coriander
- ½ teaspoon ground allspice
- ½ teaspoon ground ginger
- ½ teaspoon dry mustard
- ½ teaspoon ground fenugreek
- ½ teaspoon freshly ground black pepper
- ¼ teaspoon ground cloves
- ¼ teaspoon ground nutmeg
- ¼ teaspoon cayenne pepper
- 1½ pounds raw shrimp, peeled and deveined
- 1 tablespoon safflower oil
- 1 yellow onion, chopped
- 1 red bell pepper, chopped
- 1 green bell pepper, chopped
- 1 small zucchini, quartered lengthwise, then sliced
- 1 small carrot, thinly sliced
- 2 garlic cloves, minced
- 1 cup vegetable broth
- 1 (15-ounce) can crushed tomatoes
- 2 cups cooked brown rice
- 2 tablespoons thinly sliced scallion (green part only)

VARIATIONS

- Substitute any type of fish, cut into chunks.

- Add 1 sweet potato, peeled and cubed, and leave out seafood for a vegetarian version.

- Serve over quinoa instead of rice.

- Double the vegetable broth and serve as a soup, without any rice.

- For extra spiciness, add more cayenne pepper, hot sauce, and/or a whole Scotch bonnet or habanero pepper when you add the tomato sauce.

- Add 1 (13.5- to 15-ounce) can coconut milk with the shrimp for a creamy version.

Parchment-Baked Salmon and Veggies

Serves 2

IN a small bowl, combine 2 tablespoons of the olive oil and the basil. Set aside.

PREHEAT the oven to 450°F. Cut two pieces of parchment paper about 18×15 inches each.

ON the middle of one piece of the parchment paper, brush 1 teaspoon of the olive oil. Add one salmon fillet. Drizzle the fillet with half the lemon juice. Sprinkle with half each of the lemon zest, dill, salt, and pepper. Spread half the sliced garlic over the seasoned fish. Cover with half each of the asparagus, carrot, snow peas, fennel, and scallion. Fold the parchment paper over the fish and vegetables to form a packet, folding in short ends first, then folding the long ends over and wrapping them underneath the packet. Put the packet on a baking sheet. Repeat with the second sheet of parchment and the remaining ingredients.

BAKE the packets for 25 minutes, or until the fish flakes easily (you can open a packet to test) or has an internal temperature of 145°F.

TO serve, put each packet on a plate. Carefully cut or tear open the parchment (the steam inside will be hot). Drizzle each with half the olive oil-basil mixture and serve.

2 tablespoons plus
2 teaspoons olive oil

2 teaspoons minced fresh basil leaves

2 (6-ounce) salmon fillets

Zest and juice of 1 lemon

½ teaspoon dried dill

¼ teaspoon sea salt

¼ teaspoon freshly ground black pepper

2 garlic cloves, thinly sliced

8 spears young (thin) asparagus, cut into 1-inch pieces

1 medium carrot, halved lengthwise and thinly sliced

½ cup snow peas, cut in half

½ cup thinly sliced fennel bulb

1 scallion, thinly sliced

VARIATIONS

- Mix the olive oil with any other fresh herb(s) you like, such as cilantro, tarragon, oregano, or mint.

- Use chicken instead of fish.

- Use any other vegetables you happen to have, such as tomatoes, zucchini, yellow squash, spinach, or green beans.

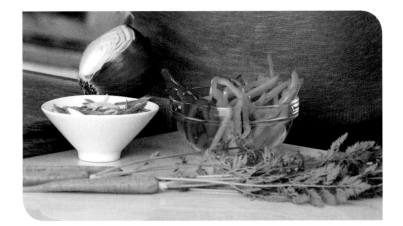

Grilled Fish Tostadas

Serves 4

PREHEAT the oven to 400°F. Cut four 12-inch squares of parchment paper.

IN the middle of each parchment square, put ¼ cup of the salsa. Top each with a fish fillet and season all the fillets with the salt and pepper. Wrap the fillets in the parchment by folding in two opposite sides of the parchment, then folding in the other two sides. Place the packets on a baking sheet, seam-side down.

ON a separate baking sheet, lay out the tortillas. Put the fish and tortillas in the oven. Bake the tortillas until crisp, about 5 minutes, flipping them halfway through. Bake the fish for 10 minutes, then carefully flip over one packet and open it. Test the fish to see if it flakes with a fork. If it does, it's done. If not, bake for 3 minutes more.

TO serve, place each tortilla on a plate. Spread the mashed avocado over the tortillas. Top with the beans. Unwrap the packets and flake one fillet over each tortilla. Top with the salsa from the packet, the shredded lettuce, and the olives and serve.

1 cup red salsa

4 (6-ounce) wild-caught white-fleshed fish fillets (halibut, tilapia, etc.)

½ teaspoon sea salt

¼ teaspoon freshly ground black pepper

8 (8-inch) sprouted-grain tortillas

2 avocados, mashed

1 cup canned black beans, drained and rinsed

1 cup shredded romaine lettuce

¼ cup chopped pitted olives

VARIATIONS

- Use shredded chicken breasts instead of the fish.

- Serve the fish over brown rice or cauliflower rice instead of tortillas.

- Spread ¼ cup fat-free refried beans over each tortilla instead of or in addition to the avocado before topping them with the fish.

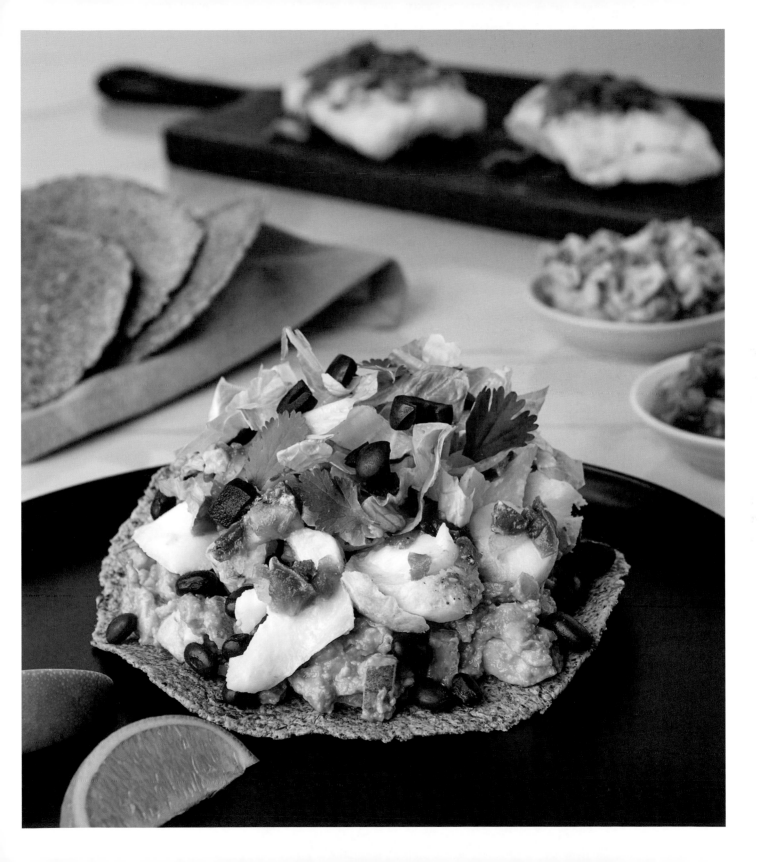

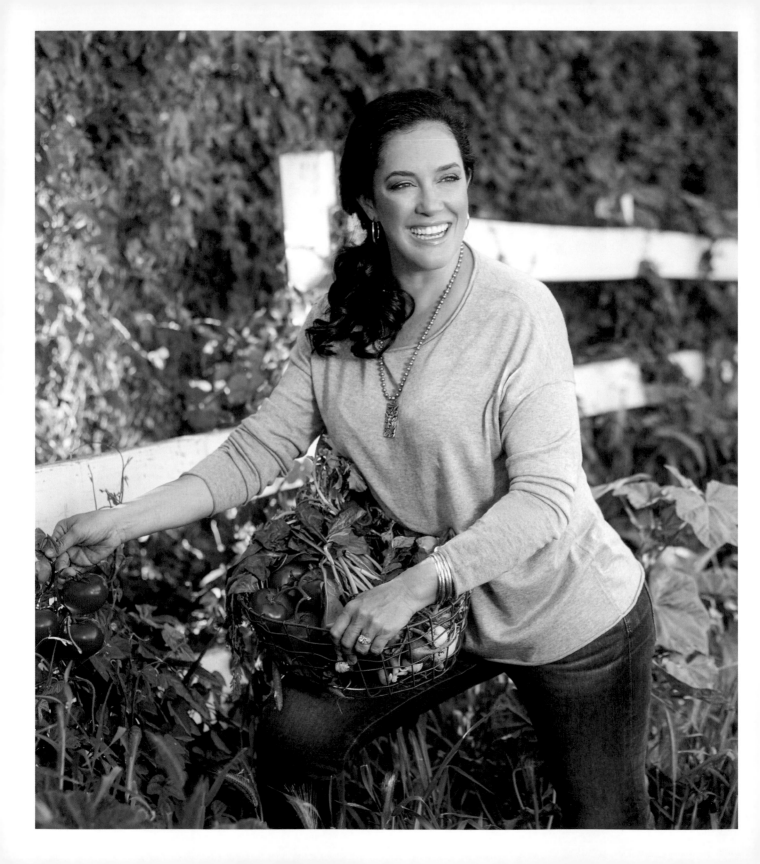

Mole Cabbage Enchiladas with Sweet Potatoes and Black Beans

Serves 8

BRING a large pot of water to a boil over high heat. Add the sweet potatoes and boil until they are soft, about 10 minutes. Scoop them out with a slotted spoon and set aside. Drop the cabbage leaves into the boiling water and blanch them for 1 minute. Remove them with tongs and put them on a plate. Set aside.

PUT all the dried chiles in a bowl and cover with boiling water (you could ladle out some of the boiling water from the potatoes and cabbage). Let them sit for 10 to 15 minutes to soften.

IN a large skillet, heat 2 tablespoons of the grapeseed oil over medium-high. Add the bell peppers and onion. Sauté until soft, about 8 minutes. Add the garlic and sauté for 2 minutes. Stir in the sweet potato cubes and beans. Transfer the mixture to a bowl and set aside.

IN the same skillet, heat 1 tablespoon of the grapeseed oil over medium heat. Drain the chilies and add them to the skillet, along with the almonds, cacao powder, sesame seeds, pumpkin seeds, paprika, oregano, xylitol (if using), coriander, cumin, cinnamon, chipotle powder, salt, pepper, and cloves. Cook for

(continued)

2 medium sweet potatoes, unpeeled, cubed

16 large green or red cabbage leaves

2 dried guajillo chiles, seeded

2 dried ancho chiles, seeded

4 tablespoons grapeseed oil

2 green bell peppers, coarsely chopped

1 medium white onion, coarsely chopped

5 garlic cloves, cut in half

1 (15-ounce) can black beans, drained and rinsed

½ cup coarsely chopped raw almonds

¼ cup raw cacao powder

2 tablespoons sesame seeds

2 tablespoons raw pumpkin seeds (pepitas)

2 tablespoons smoked paprika

2 tablespoons dried Mexican oregano

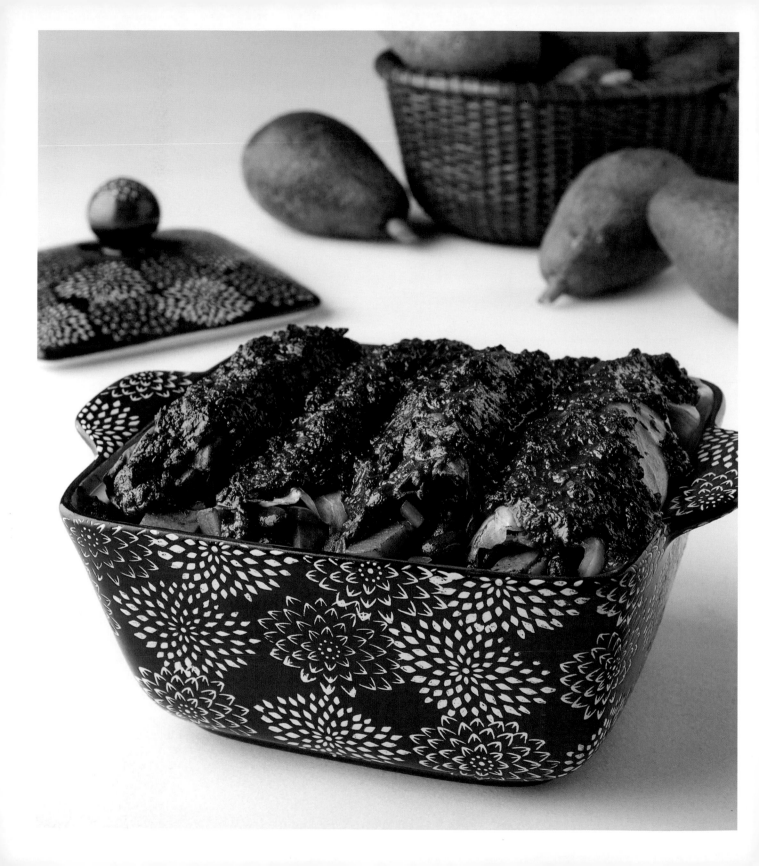

2 tablespoons xylitol
(optional)

1 tablespoon ground
coriander

1 teaspoon ground cumin

1 teaspoon ground cinnamon

1 teaspoon chipotle powder

1 teaspoon sea salt

½ teaspoon freshly ground
black pepper

¼ teaspoon ground cloves

1 (14- to 15-ounce) can
fire-roasted tomatoes

¼ cup apple cider vinegar

½ cup pitted fresh or thawed
frozen black cherries

1 bunch fresh cilantro,
leaves coarsely chopped

1 large avocado, cubed

5 minutes more, stirring continuously to toast the nuts and seeds and coat everything with the spices. Add the tomatoes and vinegar and stir, scraping up any stuck bits from the bottom of the pan. Stir in the cherries. Remove from the heat and carefully transfer the contents of the pan to a blender. Blend for 5 minutes, or until completely smooth.

IN the same skillet, heat the remaining 1 tablespoon grapeseed oil over medium heat. Return the sauce to the skillet. Bring the sauce to a simmer, then reduce the heat to low and cover the pan. Simmer for 30 to 45 minutes, checking frequently and adding water (¼ cup at a time) if the sauce starts to look too thick or dry. (It should be the consistency of a smooth tomato sauce.)

PREHEAT the oven to 400°F. Line a baking pan or casserole dish with parchment paper.

LAY out the cabbage leaves on a work surface. Divide the mixture between the cabbage leaves and roll each one up, tucking in the ends. Put the enchiladas in a casserole or shallow serving dish. Pour the mole sauce over the top, covering all the enchiladas. Bake for 20 minutes. Remove from the oven and garnish with cilantro and avocado. Serve each person two enchiladas.

VARIATIONS

- Make this recipe with warmed sprouted-grain tortillas instead of cabbage leaves.
- Add cooked shredded turkey or chicken to each enchilada in place of the black beans.

Brazilian Fish Stew

Serves 4

NOTE: You can use chilled full-fat coconut milk instead of coconut cream. Refrigerate the can of coconut milk overnight. Open the can and scoop out just the solid coconut cream (save the coconut milk for a smoothie).

PLACE the fish in a medium bowl. Drizzle with the lime juice. In a small bowl, mix together the coriander, ginger, garlic, cumin, paprika, salt, pepper, and allspice. Sprinkle the spice mixture over the fish and toss to coat. Set aside.

IN a large skillet, heat the olive oil over medium-high heat. Add the onion and sauté until very soft, about 8 minutes. Add the bell peppers and sauté for 5 minutes more. Stir in the tomatoes and tomato paste. Bring the mixture to a simmer, then add the fish and all the spice mixture and stir. Bring the stew back to a simmer, then reduce the heat to medium-low and cook, stirring occasionally, for 10 minutes. Remove the pan from the heat and add the coconut cream and xylitol (if using). Stir until the coconut cream is melted and completely combined.

TO serve, divide the quinoa among four bowls. Ladle the stew over the quinoa and top with the cilantro.

VARIATIONS

- Substitute shrimp and scallops or any other seafood combination for the salmon and haddock or cod.
- Serve over brown rice instead of quinoa.
- Omit the coconut cream and xylitol for a brothier, more savory soup.

12 ounces boneless, skinless salmon, chopped into chunks

12 ounces boneless, skinless haddock or cod, chopped into chunks

Juice of 1 lime

1 tablespoon ground coriander

1 tablespoon minced fresh ginger

2 garlic cloves, minced

½ teaspoon ground cumin

½ teaspoon paprika

½ teaspoon sea salt

½ teaspoon freshly ground black pepper

¼ teaspoon ground allspice

2 tablespoons olive oil

1 yellow onion, chopped

1 red bell pepper, chopped

1 yellow bell pepper, chopped

1 (14-ounce) can fire-roasted tomatoes

1 tablespoon tomato paste

½ cup unsweetened coconut cream (see Note)

1 tablespoon xylitol (optional)

2 cups cooked tricolor (or any color) quinoa

½ cup chopped fresh cilantro leaves

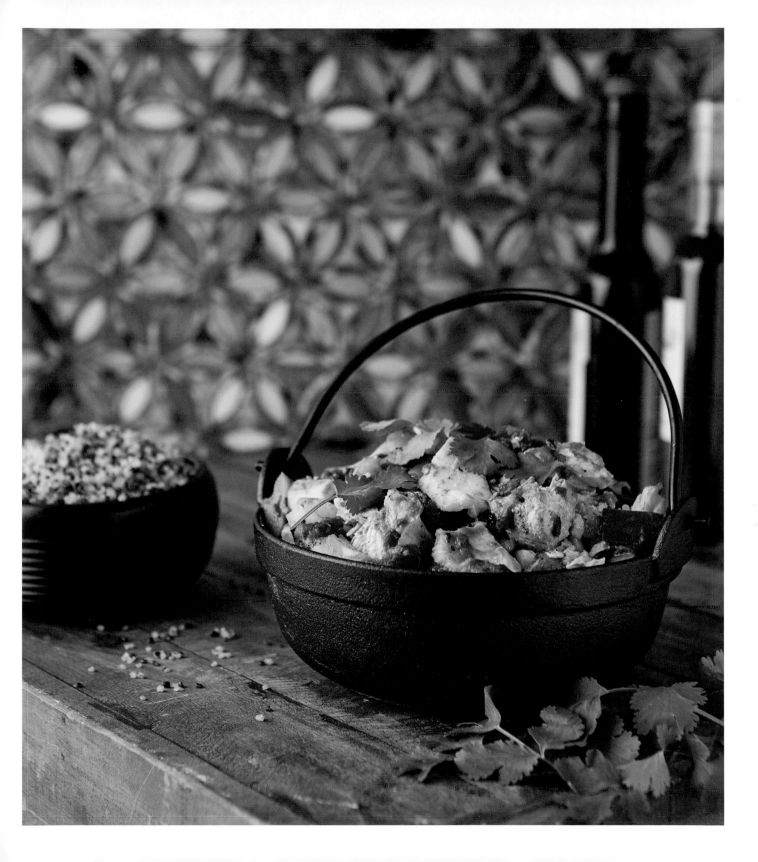

Mediterranean Veggie Burgers with Aioli Slaw

Serves 4

LAY out the shredded zucchini on a paper towel and salt it lightly. Cover with another paper towel and let sit for 5 minutes, then press to extract as much liquid as you can.

IN a large skillet, heat the olive oil over medium heat. Add the bell pepper and mushrooms. Sauté until soft, about 5 minutes. Add the zucchini and sauté for 3 minutes more. Add the garlic and scallions and sauté for 2 minutes more. Remove the pan from the heat and set aside.

IN a food processor, combine the chickpeas and oats and pulse to chop them up but not puree them. Scrape down the sides. Add the vegetable mixture and pulse to combine. Scoop everything into a large bowl. Add the eggs, olives, tahini, ¾ teaspoon of the salt, the oregano, rosemary, and red pepper flakes. Stir until everything is completely combined. Cover and refrigerate for at least 30 minutes (or overnight).

PREHEAT the oven to 375°F. Line a baking sheet with parchment paper.

IN a large bowl, combine the cabbage, mayonnaise, lemon juice, parsley, garlic powder, and remaining ¼ teaspoon salt. Stir until everything is completely combined.

TAKE the chickpea mixture out of the refrigerator. Using your hands, form the chickpea mixture into four patties and put them on the prepared baking sheet. Bake until they look golden brown and crispy, about 40 minutes, flipping them carefully halfway through.

1 medium zucchini, shredded

1 teaspoon sea salt, plus more as needed

1 tablespoon olive oil

1 red bell pepper, finely chopped

8 ounces cremini or baby bella mushrooms, finely chopped

3 garlic cloves, minced

2 scallions, minced

1 (15-ounce) can chickpeas, drained and rinsed

1 cup old-fashioned oats

2 large eggs, lightly beaten

2 tablespoons finely chopped pitted kalamata olives

1 tablespoon tahini

½ teaspoon dried oregano, crumbled

½ teaspoon dried rosemary, crumbled

½ teaspoon red pepper flakes

1 cup finely shredded cabbage

¼ cup safflower mayonnaise

1 tablespoon fresh lemon juice

1 tablespoon minced fresh flat-leaf parsley leaves

½ teaspoon garlic powder

4 slices sprouted-grain bread

½ small red onion, thinly sliced

MEANWHILE, toast the bread.

PUT a veggie burger on each slice of toast and top with the red onion and the cabbage mixture. Serve open-faced.

VARIATIONS

- Fry the veggie burgers in olive oil rather than baking them.
- Serve them on sprouted-grain or gluten-free buns.
- Serve the patties on a bed of leafy greens or steamed kale—no bread required.

Quinoa and White Bean "Meatball" Marinara

Serves 4

MAKE the marinara: In a large skillet, heat the olive oil over medium-high heat. Add the onion and carrot. Sauté until soft, about 5 minutes. Add the basil, garlic, and oregano. Sauté for 2 minutes more. Add the tomatoes, tomato paste, vinegar, and water. Bring the mixture to a simmer, then lower the heat to medium-low. Simmer for 40 minutes. If it gets too dry, add more water.

MAKE the meatballs: Preheat the oven to 375°F. Line a rimmed baking sheet with parchment paper.

IN a large skillet, heat the olive oil over medium-high heat. Add the onion, bell pepper, and carrot. Sauté until the onion softens, about 5 minutes. Add the garlic and sauté for 2 minutes more. Add the mushrooms, kale, oregano, parsley, and thyme. Cook until the mushrooms and kale shrink down, about 5 minutes. Remove from the heat and scrape the mixture into a food processor.

ADD the beans to the food processor and pulse until the beans and vegetables are chopped and well combined but not pureed. Transfer the bean mixture to a large bowl and add the quinoa, chickpea flour, nutritional yeast, salt, and pepper. Mix until everything is combined. Taste and add more salt if needed.

SHAPE the bean mixture into 24 balls and put them on the prepared baking sheet, about an inch apart. Bake for 30 minutes, or until they turn golden brown, turning them about halfway through the cooking time.

Marinara

1 tablespoon olive oil

1 medium yellow onion, finely chopped

1 small carrot, grated

¼ cup finely chopped fresh basil leaves

2 garlic cloves, minced

1 teaspoon dried oregano

1 (28-ounce) can crushed tomatoes

1 tablespoon tomato paste

1 tablespoon red wine vinegar or balsamic vinegar

1 cup water

Meatballs

2 tablespoons olive oil

1 small yellow onion, finely chopped

½ red bell pepper, finely chopped

½ small carrot, grated

3 garlic cloves, minced

8 ounces white mushrooms, finely chopped

3 cups finely chopped stemmed kale

2 teaspoons dried oregano

2 teaspoons dried parsley

½ teaspoon dried thyme

1 (15-ounce) can cannellini beans, drained and rinsed

1 cup cooked quinoa

½ cup chickpea flour

2 tablespoons nutritional yeast

½ teaspoon sea salt, plus more if needed

½ teaspoon freshly ground black pepper

¼ cup chopped fresh flat-leaf parsley leaves, for garnish

WHEN the meatballs are done, let them cool for about 10 minutes, then carefully put them into the simmering marinara sauce and stir to coat. Spoon the meatballs and sauce into four bowls and garnish with the parsley.

VARIATIONS

- Serve the meatballs over brown rice pasta or chickpea pasta (or any pasta, as long as it is wheat-free and corn-free).

- Make a meatball sub by stuffing these into a sprouted-grain roll. Sprinkle some nutritional yeast on top for a hint of "cheesiness."

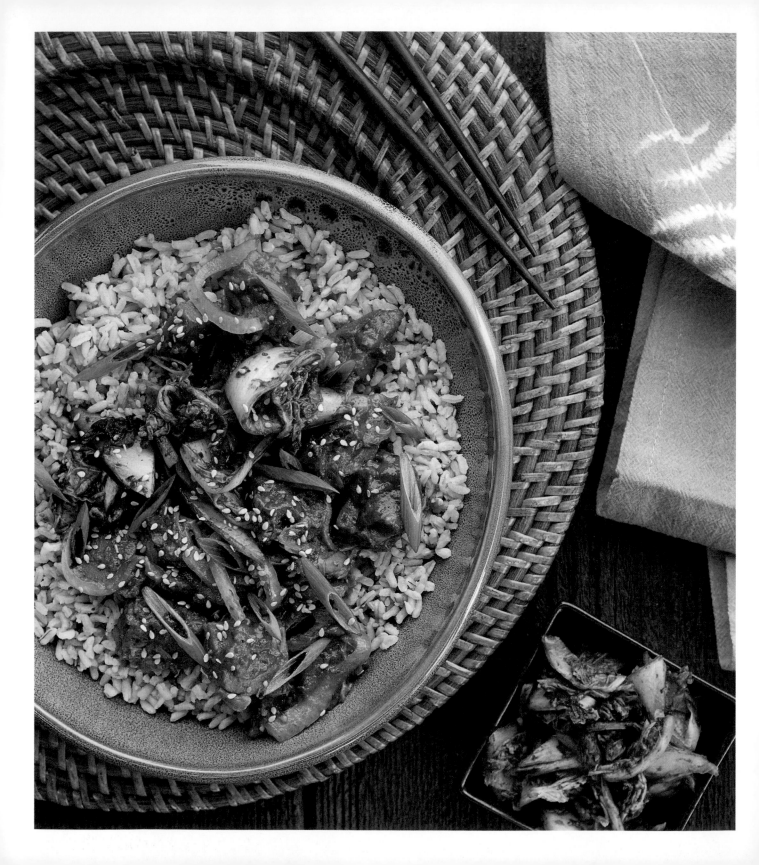

Korean BBQ Bowl with Jackfruit and Rhubarb Sauce

Serves 4

PREHEAT the oven to 400°F.

IN a medium skillet, heat the olive oil over medium-high heat. When the oil is hot, add the onion and sauté until soft, about 5 minutes. Add the garlic and sauté for 2 minutes. Add the jackfruit and sauté for 1 minute. Add the broth and cook for 5 minutes more. Stir in the BBQ sauce.

TO serve, divide the rice among four bowls. Top with the jackfruit, scallions, and sesame seeds.

VARIATIONS

- Of course you could make this with shredded pork or beef instead of jackfruit.
- You could substitute your favorite no-sugar-added BBQ sauce.

1 tablespoon olive oil

½ yellow onion, sliced

3 garlic cloves, minced

About 15 to 20 ounces shredded unflavored young jackfruit (frozen, canned, or vacuum-packed)

¼ cup vegetable broth

¾ cup Rhubarb BBQ Sauce (page 268)

2 cups cooked brown jasmine rice

½ cup thinly sliced scallions

4 teaspoons sesame seeds

Lentil Sweet Potato Curry

Serves 4

IN a large skillet, heat the grapeseed oil over medium heat. Add the onion and sauté for 5 minutes. Add the garlic and sauté for 2 minutes more. Stir in the garam masala, red pepper flakes, coriander, cumin, and turmeric. Sauté, stirring continuously, for 2 minutes. Add the sweet potatoes and cauliflower and stir to coat them with the spices. Add the broth, lentils, salt, and black pepper. Bring the curry to a boil, then lower the heat to medium-low and simmer until the lentils are soft, about 40 minutes. Remove from the heat and stir in the lemon juice. To serve, ladle the curry over the rice and sprinkle the scallion on the top.

VARIATION

• Instead of or in addition to the lentils, add 1 pound boneless, skinless chicken breasts or thighs, cut into bite-size pieces, or 1 pound raw shrimp, peeled and deveined, when you add the onions.

1 tablespoon grapeseed oil

1 medium yellow onion, coarsely chopped

6 garlic cloves, minced

2 teaspoons garam masala

1 teaspoon red pepper flakes

1 teaspoon ground coriander

1 teaspoon ground cumin

1 teaspoon ground turmeric

2 sweet potatoes, quartered lengthwise then sliced

1 head purple cauliflower, cut into florets

4 cups vegetable broth

1 cup dried green lentils

1 teaspoon sea salt

½ teaspoon freshly ground black pepper

Juice of 1 lemon

4 cups brown basmati rice

2 tablespoons thinly sliced scallion

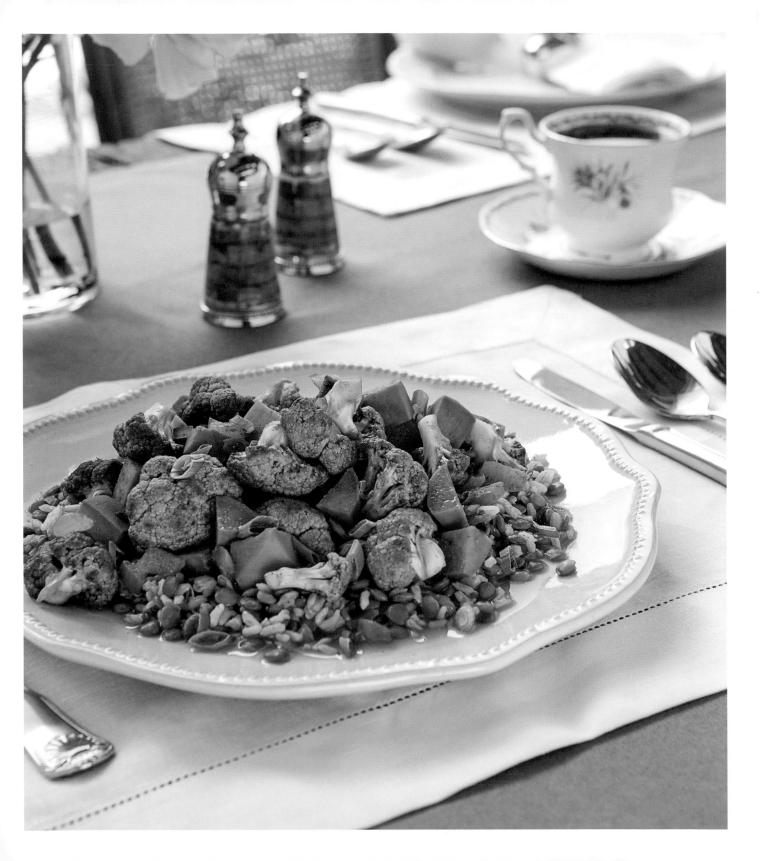

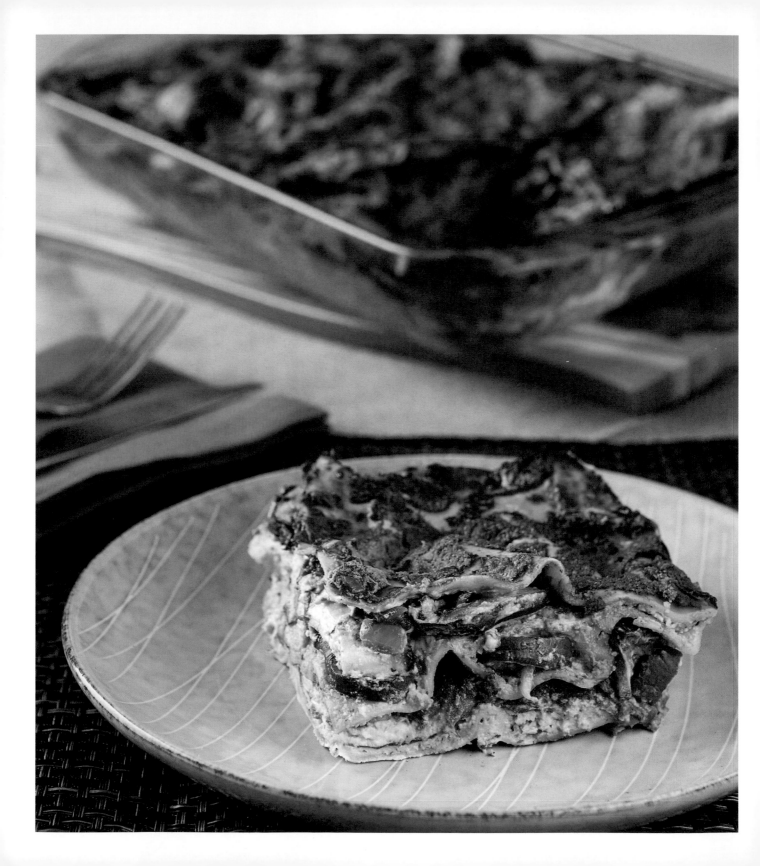

Vegetarian Baked Lasagna

Serves 6

NOTE: The night before you make this recipe, soak 2 cups raw cashews in fresh water in a covered jar. Before using them for this recipe, drain and rinse them in a strainer. You will be using half for the "ricotta" and half for the white sauce. You can also make any or all of the components of this recipe ahead of time, to make this recipe quicker to assemble.

MAKE the tomato sauce: In a medium skillet, heat the olive oil over medium heat. When it is hot, add the onion. Sauté for 3 minutes. Add the garlic and sauté for 2 minutes more. Add the tomato paste, basil, and parsley and stir to combine. Add the tomatoes, oregano, salt, and pepper. Reduce the heat to low, cover, and simmer for 30 minutes.

MAKE the ricotta: In a food processor, combine the cashews, nutritional yeast, olive oil, lemon juice, basil, garlic, oregano, salt, and pepper. Pulse to chop everything and combine. With the motor running, add the milk 1 tablespoon at a time and process until the ricotta is smooth. Set aside.

MAKE the white sauce: In a blender, combine the milk, cashews, nutritional yeast, tahini, olive oil, arrowroot mixture, garlic, and salt and blend until smooth. Pour the mixture into a small saucepan and heat over medium-low, stirring often, until the sauce begins to thicken. Remove from the heat and set aside.

ASSEMBLE the lasagna: Preheat the oven to 400°F.

(continued)

Tomato Sauce

1 tablespoon olive oil

½ sweet onion, finely chopped

2 garlic cloves, minced

2 tablespoons tomato paste

2 tablespoons minced fresh basil leaves

2 tablespoons minced fresh flat-leaf parsley

1 (15-ounce) can crushed tomatoes

1 tablespoon dried oregano

1 teaspoon sea salt

1 teaspoon freshly ground black pepper

Cashew "Ricotta"

1 cup raw cashews, soaked for at least 6 hours or overnight and drained

¼ cup nutritional yeast

1 tablespoon olive oil

1 tablespoon fresh lemon juice

4 fresh basil leaves

1 garlic clove, minced

½ teaspoon dried oregano

½ teaspoon sea salt

¼ teaspoon freshly ground black pepper

¼ cup unsweetened cashew, almond, rice, or oat milk (you may need a little more or a little less)

White Sauce

1 cup unsweetened cashew, almond, rice, or oat milk

1 cup cashews, soaked for at least 6 hours or overnight and drained

¼ cup nutritional yeast

2 tablespoons tahini or cashew butter

1 tablespoon olive oil

1 tablespoon arrowroot powder, mixed with 1 teaspoon water

1 garlic clove, minced

1 teaspoon sea salt

To Assemble

1 medium zucchini, thinly sliced

2 teaspoons sea salt

1 tablespoon olive oil

1 red bell pepper, cut into small cubes

1 cup sliced portobello mushrooms

4 cups baby spinach

1 (8- to 10-ounce) box no-boil/oven-ready gluten-free lasagna noodles (there are a variety of types available)

½ cup nutritional yeast

LAY the zucchini slices out on a paper towel and sprinkle the salt over them (this will help draw out excess liquid).

MEANWHILE, in a large skillet, heat the olive oil over medium-high heat. When it is hot, add the bell pepper and mushrooms. Sauté for 5 minutes, or until the mushrooms just begin to shrink. Transfer them to a plate and add the zucchini to the pan. Sauté until just tender, about 3 minutes. Add the spinach and sauté for 2 minutes. Remove the pan from the heat.

LINE a 9-inch square baking pan with parchment paper. Ladle in one-quarter of the tomato sauce and spread it around. Layer the remaining ingredients in this order:

   A layer of lasagna noodles

   Half the ricotta, spread over the noodles

   All the spinach and zucchini, spread evenly over the ricotta

   Half the white sauce, poured over the spinach and zucchini

   One-third of the remaining tomato sauce

   A second layer of lasagna noodles

   The remaining ricotta, spread over the noodles

   The bell pepper–mushroom mixture, evenly spread over the ricotta

   The remaining white sauce, poured over the peppers and mushrooms

   Half the remaining tomato sauce

   A third layer of lasagna noodles

   The remaining tomato sauce

TOP the lasagna evenly with the nutritional yeast. Cover the pan with aluminum foil and bake for 45 minutes. Remove the foil and bake for 10 minutes more. Remove the pan from the oven and let the lasagna sit for 15 minutes before serving.

CUT the lasagna into six squares and scoop each out carefully to serve.

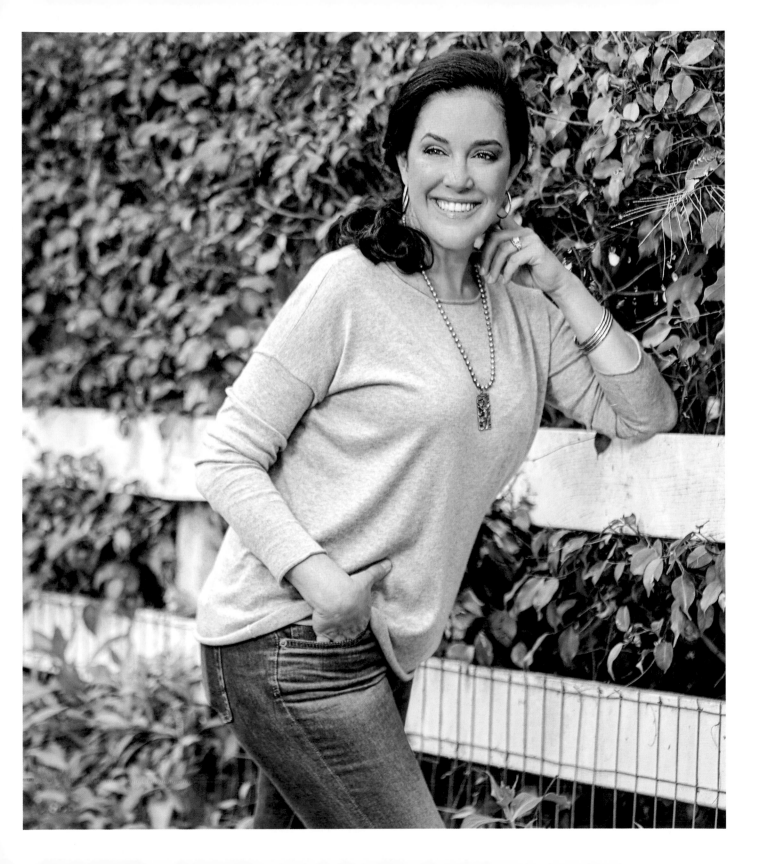

SNACKS

Grilled Mushroom Skewers with Balsamic Glaze

Serves 4

IN a zip-top plastic bag, combine the vinegar, tamari, garlic, basil, rosemary, and pepper. Put the mushrooms in the marinade and seal the bag. Tilt it a few times to coat the mushrooms. Marinate at room temperature for at least 30 minutes or overnight in the refrigerator. Soak 8 wooden skewers in water for 30 minutes.

PREHEAT a grill to medium-high heat, or preheat the broiler.

SKEWER 6 mushroom halves on each skewer, reserving the marinade. Grill or broil the mushrooms until they start to look crispy and charred, about 4 minutes each side (be careful not to burn them). Transfer the mushrooms to a platter and drizzle with the marinade. Serve two skewers per person.

¼ cup balsamic vinegar

1 tablespoon tamari or coconut aminos

4 garlic cloves, minced

1 teaspoon minced fresh basil leaves

½ teaspoon minced fresh rosemary

¼ teaspoon freshly ground black pepper

24 cremini or baby bella mushrooms, cut in half

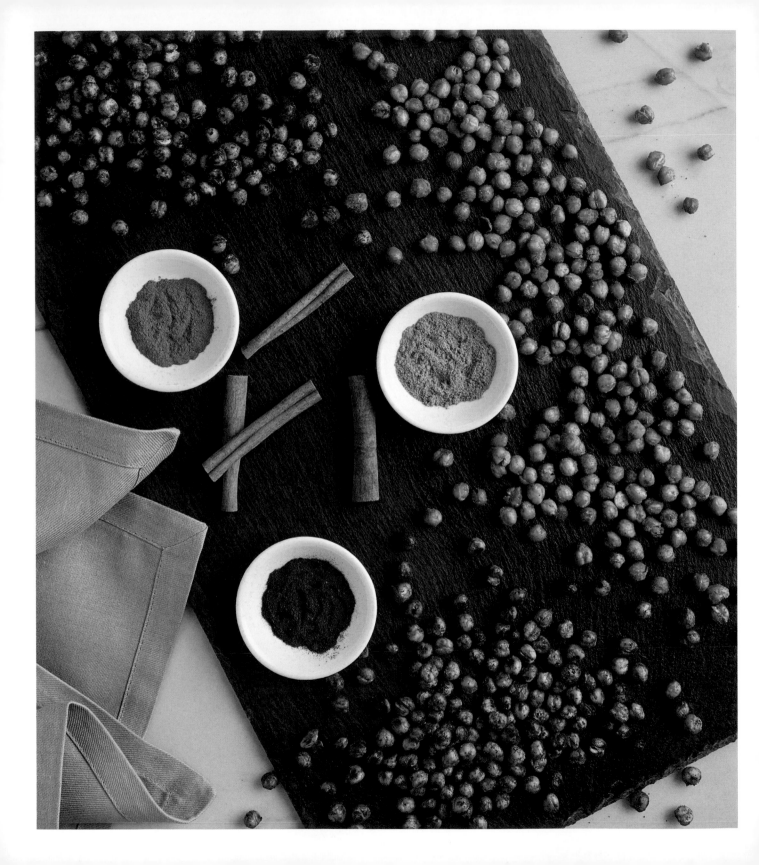

Three-Way Roasted Chickpeas

Serves 4

PREHEAT the oven to 375°F. Line a rimmed baking sheet with parchment paper.

IN a medium bowl, add all the seasonings for whichever flavor you want to make. Add the chickpeas and toss to coat.

PUT the chickpeas on the prepared baking sheet, spreading them out evenly. Bake, stirring occasionally, for 40 to 45 minutes, or until the chickpeas are crispy. Store the chickpeas in an airtight container at room temperature for up to 3 days.

1 cup chickpeas, drained and rinsed

For Cinnamon Chickpeas

2 teaspoons xylitol

1 teaspoon ground cinnamon

¼ teaspoon sea salt

For Curry Chickpeas

½ teaspoon curry powder

¼ teaspoon ground turmeric

¼ teaspoon sea salt

⅛ teaspoon red pepper flakes

For Red Hot Chili Chickpeas

½ teaspoon paprika (regular or smoked)

½ teaspoon sea salt

¼ teaspoon chili powder

¼ teaspoon ground cumin

¼ teaspoon cayenne pepper

Spicy Salmon Jerky

Makes 4 servings

IN a wide glass or plastic container, combine the tamari, coconut aminos, lemon juice, pepper, liquid smoke, stevia, and hot sauce. Slice the salmon fillets lengthwise into ¼-inch-thick slices. Place the salmon in the marinade, making sure every piece is coated. Cover the bowl and refrigerate for 4 hours.

PREHEAT the oven to 200°F. Line a large rimmed baking sheet with parchment paper and place a wire rack on top of the parchment.

ARRANGE the salmon pieces on the rack in a single layer, leaving a bit of space between them. Bake for 3 hours, until the jerky is dry and leathery but still flexible. Remove from the oven and let cool completely.

TRANSFER the jerky to an airtight container and refrigerate for up to 2 weeks; freeze for up to 3 months.

1 cup tamari

2 tablespoons coconut aminos

2 tablespoons fresh lemon juice

1½ tablespoons freshly ground black pepper

2 teaspoons liquid smoke flavoring

20 to 30 drops stevia

12 dashes of hot sauce (such as Tabasco), or more to taste

1½ pounds salmon fillets, skin removed

Slow Cooker Baked Apples

Serves 4

IN a medium bowl, mix together the apricots, oats, ¼ cup of the pecans, the almond butter, xylitol (if using), cinnamon, ginger, and salt.

CUT the tops off the apples. Scoop or cut out the core (a melon baller works well for this), but leave the bottom ½ inch of the apples intact. Fill the apples with the apricot mixture. Put them in a slow cooker with ¼ cup water. Cover and cook on high for 2 hours or on low for 4 hours, until the apples are soft and easily pierced with a fork.

TRANSFER the apples to individual dessert plates or bowls and top with whipped cream. Sprinkle evenly with the remaining 1 tablespoon pecans and dust with cinnamon, then serve.

4 apricots, pitted and finely chopped

⅓ cup old-fashioned oats

¼ cup plus 1 tablespoon chopped pecans

¼ cup almond butter

2 tablespoons xylitol (optional)

1 teaspoon ground cinnamon, plus more for garnish

¼ teaspoon ground ginger

¼ teaspoon sea salt

4 apples

Coconut Whipped Cream (page 266)

Chocolate-Orange Power Balls

Makes 16 (2 balls per serving)

IN a food processor, puree the apricots. And the nut butter, cacao powder, chia seeds, orange zest, mint extract, vanilla, and salt. Process until smooth and fully combined. Add the cacao nibs and pulse a few times to combine but not enough to puree them.

LINE a baking sheet that will fit in your freezer with parchment paper. Put the chopped almonds on a plate.

SCOOP tablespoons of the mixture and roll them into balls with your hands. Roll them in the almonds to coat and put them on the prepared baking sheet. Freeze the balls overnight, then transfer them to an airtight container or zip-top bag and freeze them for a quick snack to grab when you are on the go. They will last about 3 months in the freezer.

1 cup chopped pitted ripe apricots

1 cup any nut butter (almond, cashew, etc.)

3 tablespoons raw cacao powder

2 tablespoons chia seeds

2 teaspoons orange zest

1 teaspoon pure mint extract

1 teaspoon pure vanilla extract

¼ teaspoon sea salt

2 tablespoons raw cacao nibs

½ cup chopped raw almonds

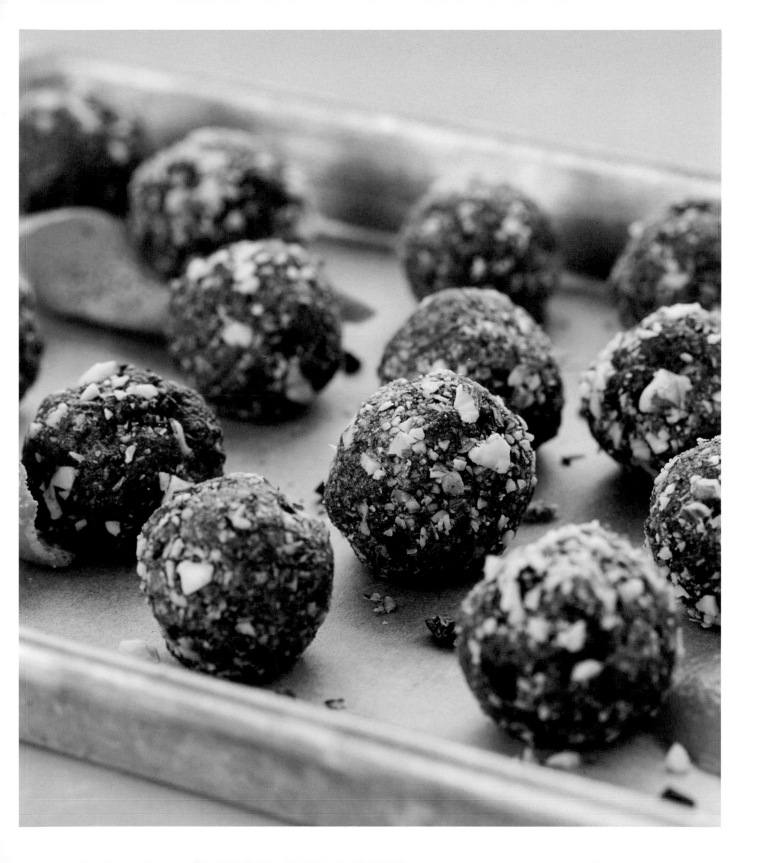

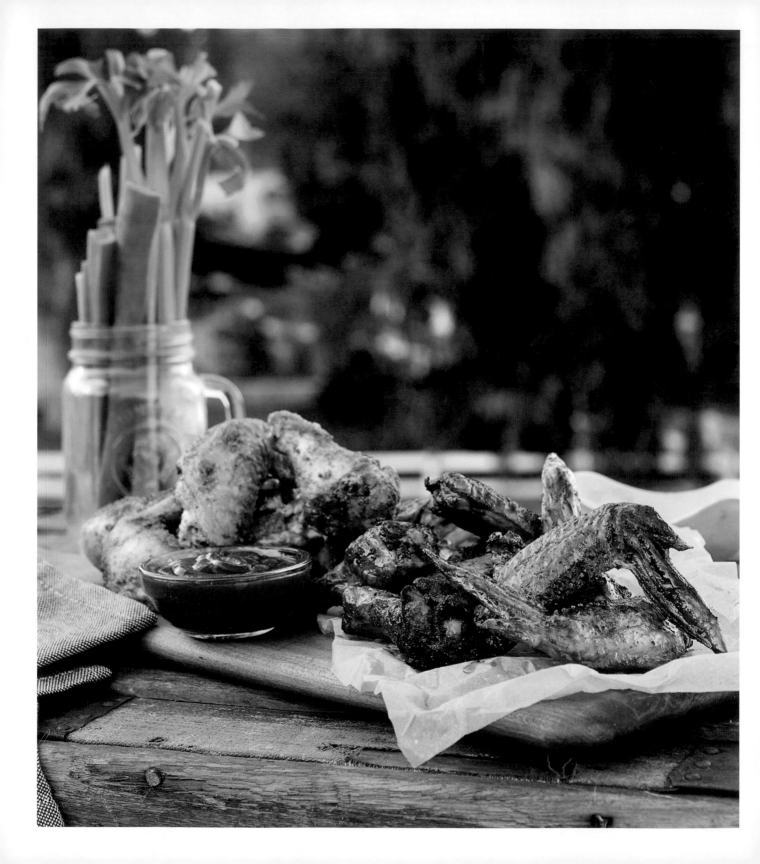

Baked Buffalo Wings, Two Ways

Makes 20 wings (4 wings per serving)

PREHEAT the oven to 400°F. Line a baking sheet with parchment paper.

TO make a "breaded" version, in a large zip-top bag, combine the flour, cayenne, garlic powder, black pepper, and salt. To make an "unbreaded" version, omit the flour.

IN a medium bowl, combine the lime juice and hot sauce.

DIP the wings in the hot sauce mixture to coat them, then drop them in the bag with the seasoning. Shake to coat the wings with the seasoning.

PUT the wings on the prepared baking sheet, spreading them out so they don't touch each other. Bake for 45 minutes, or until the wings look crispy, turning them once halfway through the cooking time.

SERVE with the celery and carrot sticks and ranch dressing alongside or with additional hot sauce.

½ cup spelt flour or other gluten-free flour (optional)

1 tablespoon cayenne pepper

1 teaspoon garlic powder

¼ teaspoon freshly ground black pepper

⅛ teaspoon sea salt

¼ cup fresh lime juice

¼ cup hot sauce (such as Tabasco or Frank's RedHot), plus more for serving, if desired

20 chicken wings

10 celery stalks, halved lengthwise

5 carrots, quartered lengthwise

Creamy Ranch Dressing (page 270)

DESSERTS

Berry Good No-Bake Cheesecake

Serves 8

REFRIGERATE the cans of coconut milk overnight. Open the cans and scoop just the solid coconut cream into a bowl (save the coconut milk for a smoothie); you need 1 cup of the coconut cream (save the rest for another use).

IN a food processor, combine the almonds, walnuts, and prunes. Pulse until the mixture resembles fine crumbs and sticks together. Divide the mixture evenly among eight 6-ounce ramekins and press it down to cover the bottom and slightly up the sides.

RINSE out the food processor bowl. In the food processor, combine the cashews, coconut solids, blueberries, blackberries, lemon zest, lemon juice, xylitol (if using), and salt. Process until smooth. Divide the mixture among the ramekins, pouring it over the crust.

PUT the ramekins in the freezer and freeze until solid, at least 6 hours or overnight.

BEFORE serving, remove the ramekins from the freezer and set aside.

IN a small saucepan, combine the orange and all its juices, raspberries, strawberries, and cranberries. Heat over medium heat, stirring frequently, until the mixture begins to simmer. Stir in the arrowroot mixture and simmer until the sauce thickens. Set aside to cool slightly, about 10 minutes.

DRIZZLE the cheesecakes with the warm fruit sauce and serve immediately.

2 or 3 (13- to 15-ounce) cans full-fat coconut milk

½ cup raw almonds

½ cup raw walnuts

1 cup prunes

2 cups raw cashews, soaked overnight, drained, and rinsed

1 cup blueberries

1 cup blackberries

Zest and juice of 1 large lemon

2 tablespoons xylitol (optional)

¼ teaspoon sea salt

1 orange, peeled, seeded, and chopped

½ cup raspberries

½ cup strawberries

¼ cup cranberries

1 tablespoon arrowroot powder, mixed with 1 tablespoon water

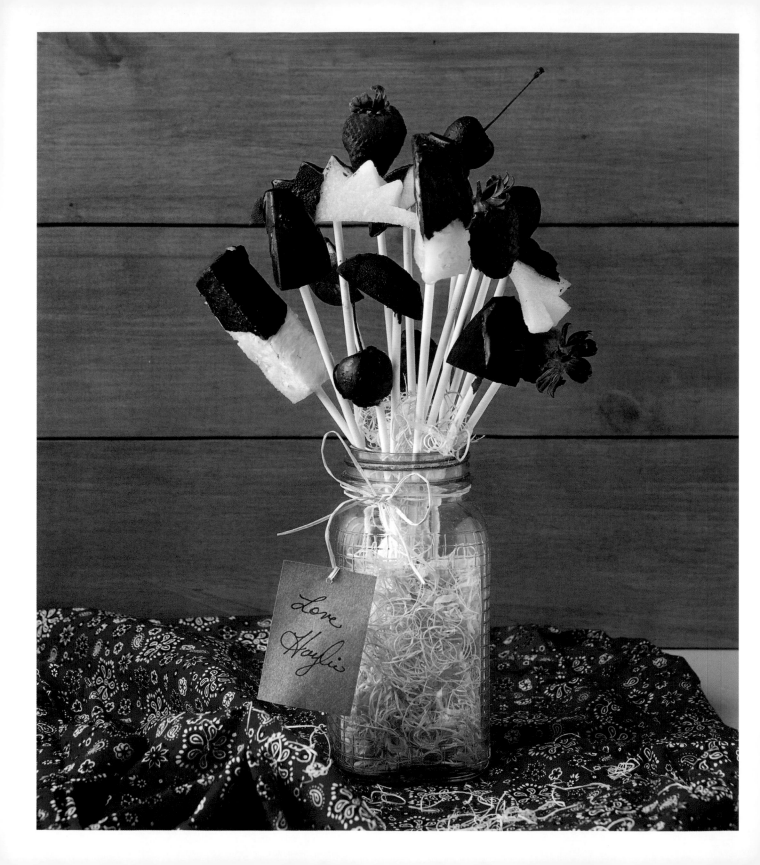

Chocolate-Dipped Salad Bar

Serves 6

IN a small saucepan, melt the coconut oil over low heat. Stir in the cacao powder.

LINE a tray that will fit into your freezer with parchment paper. Spear each of your fruit and vegetable chunks with a cake pop stick. Dip them into the chocolate to coat and put them on the parchment paper. Freeze until the chocolate is firm, 20 to 30 minutes.

1 tablespoon coconut oil

⅓ cup raw cacao powder

12 chunks of assorted fruits and vegetables such as:

Whole strawberries

Pineapple spears

Peach slices

Radishes

Jicama, cut into any shape

Pineapple "Push-Up" Pops

Serves 7

LINE seven wells of a muffin tin with paper liners.

PUREE the pineapple and coconut milk in a blender until smooth. Stir in the cacao nibs. Pour the pineapple mixture into the prepared muffin cups, dividing it evenly. Cover with plastic wrap, then stick ice pop sticks through the plastic into the center of each cup (the plastic wrap helps the sticks stay upright as the pops freeze). Freeze overnight.

TO serve, remove the plastic wrap, lift out the pops, peel off the paper liners, and enjoy immediately.

1 whole pineapple, peeled, cored, and cut into chunks (about 3 cups)

¾ cup canned coconut milk (not low-fat)

¼ cup raw cacao nibs

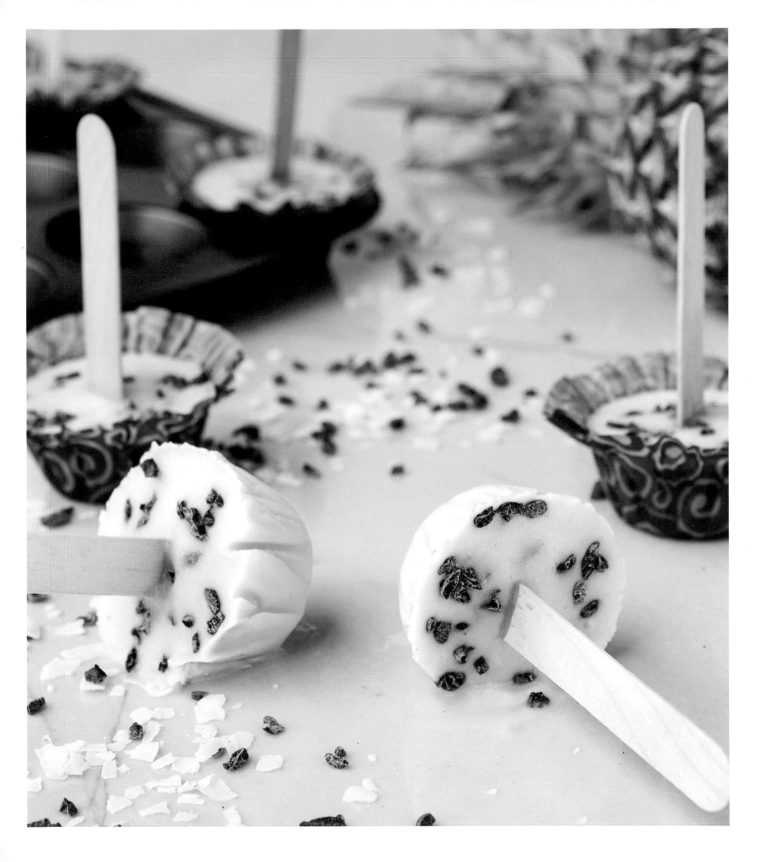

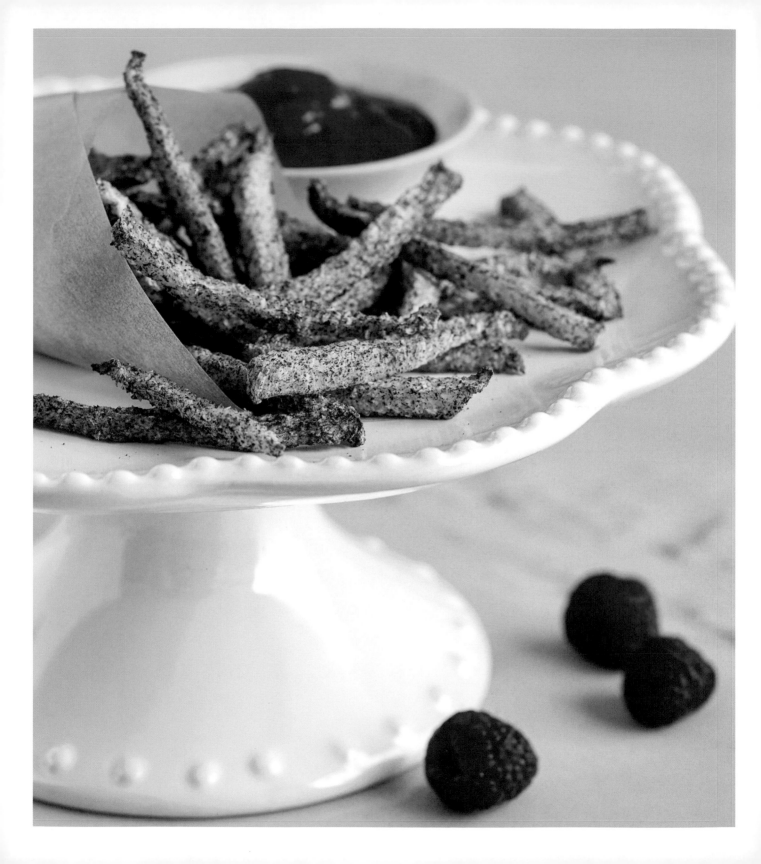

Cinnamon Jicama Fries with Raspberry Dipping Sauce

Serves 2 (but vegetables are unlimited)

1 tablespoon ground cinnamon

1 medium jicama, peeled and cut into fry shapes

1 pint raspberries

Juice of ½ lime

PREHEAT the oven to 300°F. Line a rimmed baking sheet with parchment paper.

PUT the cinnamon in a gallon-size zip-top bag. Add the jicama, seal, and shake to coat. Put the jicama fries on the baking sheet, spread out so they aren't touching. Bake for 35 minutes, or until the fries look crispy.

MEANWHILE, puree the raspberries and lime juice in a blender, then warm the puree in a small saucepan over low heat.

SERVE the hot fries with the raspberry dipping sauce.

DIY STAPLE FOODS
AND CONDIMENTS

Coconut Sour Cream

Makes about ½ cup

REFRIGERATE the can of coconut milk overnight. Open the can and scoop just the solid coconut cream into a medium bowl (save the coconut milk for a smoothie). Add the lemon juice and salt and whisk until combined. Taste and season with more salt and lemon juice, if desired. Cover and refrigerate for about 1 hour before serving to allow the flavors to combine. Depending on the coconut milk you buy, your sour cream might end up a little grainier than dairy sour cream. You can also strain it through a fine-mesh sieve if you want it extra smooth. The sour cream will keep in an airtight container in the refrigerator for up to 2 days.

1 (15-ounce) can full-fat coconut milk

1 tablespoon fresh lemon juice, plus more if needed

⅛ teaspoon sea salt, plus more if needed

Cashew Sour Cream

Makes about 1 cup

DRAIN and rinse the cashews, and put them in a food processor. Add the water, lemon juice, vinegar, and salt. Process until everything is smooth and creamy, about 5 minutes, scraping down the sides every minute or so. If it seems too thick, add more water, a tablespoon at a time.

TRANSFER the sour cream to an airtight container and refrigerate for at least 1 hour or up to overnight before serving. It will get thicker as it chills. The sour cream will keep in the refrigerator for up to 5 days.

1 cup raw cashews, soaked in water for at least 3 hours or overnight

½ cup spring water

Juice of ½ lemon

½ teaspoon white wine vinegar or apple cider vinegar

½ teaspoon sea salt

Shreddable Sliceable Cashew Cheese

Makes about 18 ounces

CHOOSE a container that can hold about 3 cups—a bowl or glass measuring cup works well. Grease it with coconut oil.

IN a blender, combine the cashews, ⅓ cup of the water, tahini, nutritional yeast, coconut oil, lemon juice, and salt. Blend until very smooth, about 5 minutes, stopping to scrape down the sides as needed. Leave this mixture in the blender.

IN a small saucepan, add the remaining 1 cup water and the agar-agar powder. Bring the mixture to a boil over high heat, stirring continuously, then boil for 1 minute (time it to be precise), as you continue to stir. Remove from the heat and pour the agar-agar mixture into the blender. Blend to combine it with the cashew mixture, about 1 minute (start on low speed so the hot mixture doesn't spatter).

IMMEDIATELY pour the mixture into the prepared container. Refrigerate until set, about 4 hours or up to overnight. To remove the cheese, turn the bowl upside down onto a plate and slice, shred, or serve as is. You can store the cheese in the refrigerator for up to 1 week.

Coconut oil, for greasing

1 cup raw cashews

1⅓ cups water

¼ cup tahini

¼ cup nutritional yeast

2 tablespoons coconut oil

1 tablespoon fresh lemon juice

2½ teaspoons sea salt

1 tablespoon agar-agar powder (not flakes)

Easy-Peasy
Nacho Cheesy

Makes about 2½ cups

IN a high-powered blender, pulse the peppers to chop them up a bit. Drain and rinse the cashews and add them to the blender. Add the nutritional yeast, green chiles, salt, garlic, mustard, turmeric, and onion powder. Blend until smooth and creamy, about 5 minutes, stopping about once every minute to scrape down the sides.

ONCE the sauce is smooth, with the blender running, drizzle in the olive oil and blend just until combined. Taste and add more salt if desired.

STORE the cheese in an airtight glass container in the fridge for up to 1 week. (If you're following the Fast Metabolism Diet, 3 tablespoons would count as a healthy-fat portion.)

1½ cups coarsely chopped orange or red bell peppers (or a combination)

1 cup raw cashews, soaked in water for at least 3 hours or overnight

¼ cup nutritional yeast

¼ cup canned green chiles

1 teaspoon sea salt

1 small garlic clove, minced

½ teaspoon dry mustard

¼ teaspoon ground turmeric

¼ teaspoon onion powder

¼ cup olive oil

Cashew Cream Cheese

Makes about 1 cup

DRAIN and rinse the cashews. Put the cashews, 1 teaspoon of lemon juice, and the salt in a food processor. Process until smooth, stopping to scrape down the sides as needed, about 5 minutes. Taste and add additional salt and/or lemon juice if you like. Add a tablespoon or two of water to thin the mixture as needed.

SERVE immediately or transfer to an airtight container and refrigerate for up to 1 week.

1 cup raw cashews, soaked in water for 4 to 8 hours or overnight

1 teaspoon fresh lemon juice, plus more as needed

½ teaspoon sea salt, plus more as needed

1 to 2 tablespoons water, as needed

Coconut Whipped Cream

Serves 4

REFRIGERATE the can of coconut milk overnight. Open the can and scoop just the solid coconut cream into a large bowl (save the coconut milk for a smoothie). Add the vanilla and stevia and beat with a handheld mixer until thick and fluffy, about 4 minutes. Use immediately.

1 (14-ounce) can coconut milk

1 teaspoon pure vanilla extract

10 drops liquid stevia, or to taste

Fire-Roasted Salsa

Makes about 1½ cups

IN a small, ungreased skillet, roast the whole jalapeños and garlic cloves over medium heat, turning them regularly, until they are soft and blotchy brown, about 10 minutes. Remove from the heat and let cool. When they are cool enough to handle, pull the stems off the peppers and peel the garlic.

PLACE the peppers and garlic in a food processor and pulse until finely chopped. Add the tomatoes with their juices. Pulse a few times to make a coarse puree.

TRANSFER the puree to a bowl. Stir in the cilantro and lime juice, and season with salt. Store covered in the refrigerator for up to 3 days.

1 or 2 whole jalapeños (or more, if you like it spicier)

3 garlic cloves, unpeeled

1 (15-ounce) can fire-roasted diced tomatoes, with their juices

½ cup loosely packed chopped fresh cilantro

2 tablespoons fresh lime juice

¼ teaspoon sea salt, or to taste

Homemade No-Sugar-Added Ketchup

Makes 2 cups

IN a medium bowl, whisk together all of the ingredients until completely blended. Cover and refrigerate for at least 2 hours or preferably overnight to let the flavors blend before serving. Store the ketchup in an airtight container in the fridge for up to 1 week.

2 (6-ounce) cans tomato paste

¼ cup apple cider vinegar

1½ teaspoons mustard (no sugar added)

¼ cup plus 2 tablespoons water

½ teaspoon sea salt

½ teaspoon ground cinnamon

¼ teaspoon garlic powder

⅛ teaspoon ground cloves

4 packets powdered stevia (about ½ teaspoon; optional)

Rhubarb BBQ Sauce

Makes 1½ cups

IN a medium saucepan, combine the rhubarb, onion, and garlic. Cook over medium heat, stirring occasionally, until the onion softens, about 5 minutes. Stir in the roasted peppers, xylitol, vinegar, lemon juice, mustard, cumin, chipotle powder, paprika, and salt, reduce the heat to medium-low, and simmer until the rhubarb is soft enough to mash with the back of a spoon, about 10 minutes. Carefully transfer the sauce to a blender and puree (or use an immersion blender to puree it right in the pot). Store in an airtight container in the refrigerator for up to 1 week.

8 ounces rhubarb (about 3 stalks), sliced

½ cup chopped onion

1 garlic clove, chopped

¼ cup jarred roasted red peppers, drained

3 tablespoons xylitol

2 tablespoons apple cider vinegar

1 teaspoon fresh lemon juice

1 teaspoon Dijon mustard (no sugar added)

½ teaspoon ground cumin

½ teaspoon chipotle powder

½ teaspoon smoked paprika

¼ teaspoon sea salt

Raspberry Vinaigrette

Makes about ¾ cup (2 to 4 tablespoons per serving)

COMBINE all the ingredients in a blender and blend until smooth. Or mash or muddle the raspberries well in the bottom of a jar, then add the remaining ingredients and shake well. Store in an airtight container in the refrigerator for up to 1 week.

1 shallot, minced

1 tablespoon Dijon mustard (no sugar added)

2 tablespoons apple cider vinegar

½ pint fresh raspberries, or about ¾ cup frozen

½ teaspoon orange zest

1 packet powdered stevia (about ⅛ teaspoon; optional)

Creamy Lemon-Herb Dressing

Makes about ¾ cup (2 to 4 tablespoons per serving)

IN a blender or food processor, combine the egg whites, lemon juice, salt, garlic powder, onion powder, and pepper. Add any add-ins of your choice (except stevia). Pulse to combine. While the blender is running, slowly add the water until the mixture reaches the desired consistency. Taste and adjust the seasonings, if needed, and add stevia, if desired. Store in an airtight container in the refrigerator for up to 1 week.

3 hard-boiled egg whites

2 tablespoons fresh lemon juice

½ teaspoon sea salt

½ teaspoon garlic powder, or 2 garlic cloves, minced

2 teaspoons onion powder

Freshly ground black pepper

¾ cup water

Add-ins
(choose one or more)

2 tablespoons chopped fresh parsley, or 2 teaspoons dried

1 tablespoon chopped fresh dill, or 1 teaspoon dried

1 tablespoon chopped fresh cilantro, or 1 teaspoon dried

1 tablespoon chopped fresh mint, or 1 teaspoon dried

1 teaspoon Dijon mustard (no sugar added), or more to taste

Stevia or xylitol

Creamy Ranch Dressing

Makes a scant 1 cup

MAKE the spice mix: Stir together all the spice mix ingredients. Set aside 2 tablespoons for the dressing and store the rest in a sealed jar or zip-top bag at room temperature.

MAKE the dressing: In a small bowl, whisk together the mayonnaise, almond milk, reserved 2 tablespoons spice mix, and the vinegar. Cover and chill for at least 2 hours or up to overnight before using. (Store in the refrigerator for up to 1 week.)

Spice Mix

¼ cup dried parsley

2 teaspoons dried dill

2 teaspoons onion powder

1½ teaspoons sea salt

1 teaspoon dried basil

1 teaspoon freshly ground black pepper

½ teaspoon garlic powder

Dressing

⅔ cup safflower mayonnaise

3 tablespoons unsweetened almond milk

¼ teaspoon white vinegar

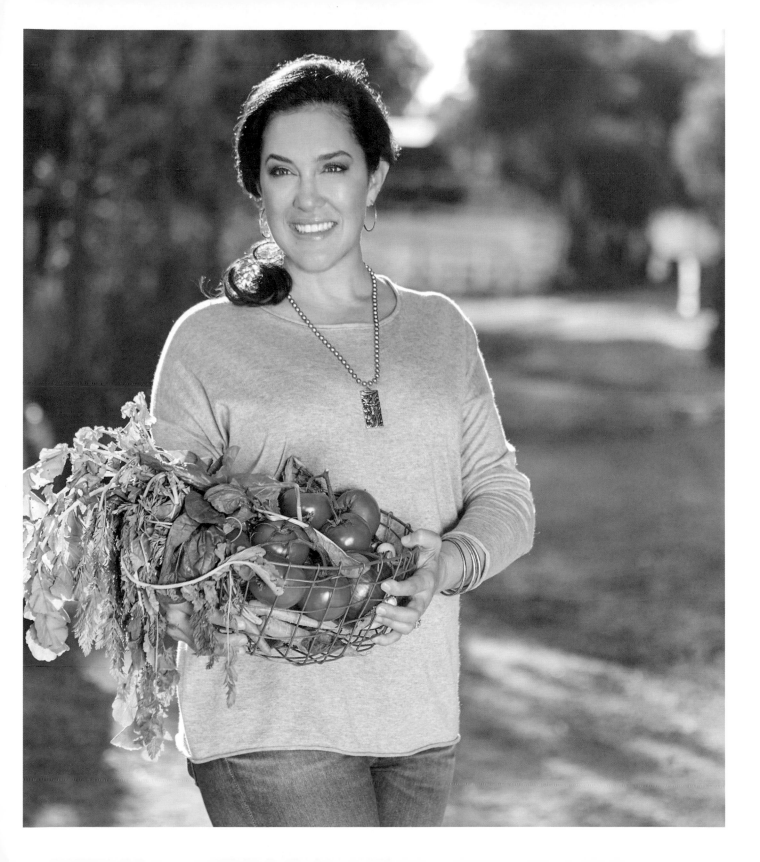

Basic Balsamic Vinaigrette

Makes about ¼ cup (2 to 4 tablespoons per serving)

BLEND, whisk, or shake everything together.

4 garlic cloves, minced

3 tablespoons balsamic vinegar

1 teaspoon dried oregano, or 1 tablespoon minced fresh oregano

1 teaspoon dried thyme, or 1 tablespoon minced fresh thyme

1 teaspoon Dijon mustard (no sugar added)

1 teaspoon freshly ground black pepper

Sesame-Ginger Dressing

Makes about ½ cup (2 to 4 tablespoons per serving)

PLACE the cashew butter in a small saucepan and gently warm it over low heat until it gets soft. Remove from the heat and add the remaining ingredients. Whisk until the mixture is smooth and creamy. Cover and chill for 30 minutes before serving, or store in an airtight container in the refrigerator for up to 1 week.

¼ cup raw cashew butter

3 tablespoons tamari

1 tablespoon red wine vinegar

2 teaspoons grated fresh ginger

1 teaspoon sesame oil

1 teaspoon olive oil

½ teaspoon sesame seeds

French Dressing

Makes about 1⅓ cups (2 to 4 tablespoons per serving)

COMBINE all the ingredients in a blender and blend until smooth. Store in an airtight container in the refrigerator for up to 1 week.

¼ cup apple cider vinegar

2 packets powdered stevia (about ¼ teaspoon)

½ cup no-sugar-added ketchup, store-bought or homemade (see page 267)

⅔ cup extra-virgin olive oil

4 teaspoons mild paprika

2 teaspoons dry mustard

½ teaspoon celery seed

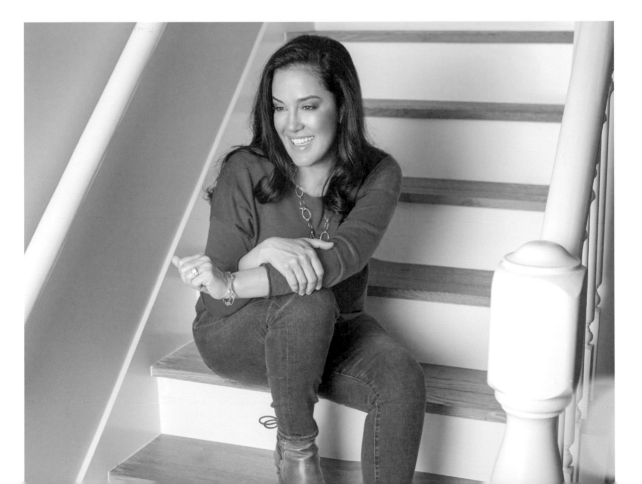

Basic Vegetable Broth

Makes about 2 quarts

PUT the vegetables in a slow cooker and sprinkle the vinegar, salt, pepper, and turmeric over them. Cover with the water. Cover and cook on low for 8 to 12 hours or on high for 4 to 6 hours.

PUT a fine-mesh strainer over a large bowl. Carefully pour the broth into the strainer. Press on the vegetables with a ladle or wooden spoon to get as much liquid out of them as you can, then discard them. Taste the broth and add more salt and pepper, if desired. Transfer the stock to airtight containers, let cool, then store in the freezer so you are always ready to make soup. It will keep in the freezer for up to 3 months.

4 cups coarsely chopped vegetables from your refrigerator or freezer (avoid broccoli, cauliflower, cabbage, and asparagus for broth, although these are good for making fresh soup), such as:

Onions, unpeeled, quartered

Leeks, trimmed, sliced

Garlic cloves

Carrots

Celery

Tomatoes

Kale

Beet greens

Bok choy

Sweet potatoes and/or their peelings

Parsnips

Turnips

Parsley

Cilantro

1 tablespoon apple cider vinegar

1 teaspoon sea salt, plus more if needed

½ teaspoon freshly ground black pepper, plus more if needed

¼ teaspoon ground turmeric

8 cups spring water

ACKNOWLEDGMENTS

The kitchen has been my pharmacy and the heart of our home. With this cookbook, my desire is to bring health, hope, and pleasure to you and your tribe through some of my most favorite dishes. This would not have been possible if not for the dedication and blind faith of many of my loved ones, colleagues, clients, community, and friends.

First, my literary agent, Alex Glass. You have taken my dreams and made them into six hardcover realities. You have been a warrior for my vision and a mentor through many diverse and wild business ventures. You have been the catalyst for changing millions of people's lives around the globe, and we are all eternally grateful to you.

Eve Adamson, I am honored to have our names together on the covers of these amazing books. You have taken my words and ideas and brought them to life so that they could touch the lives of so many.

I am also deeply grateful to our new team at Houghton Mifflin Harcourt: Deb Brody, Olivia Bartz, Tai Blanche, Rita Sowen, and Brianna Yamashita, thank you for taking this cookbook to the next level.

Bob Marty, my Public Television guru, thank you for spearheading this significant piece of our outreach. This has been an amazing opportunity to have the tools and resources available to those who are ready to change their lives! Melanie Parish, my coach of a million years, thank you for believing in me and pushing me further that I thought possible. Marc Chaplin, my legal pillar, your guidance has been and will continue to be invaluable to my business and my life. To the Lanham family and the Watkins Family, you have been both friends and mentors throughout my life and have inspired me and supported me relentlessly, I thank you.

To Steve Tully, Leilani Roh, John Tillotson, Shelley Edgerton, Alicia Freeman, Hanna Allman, Marq Deas, Katie Lanham, Eiland Pomroy, Gracen Pomroy, and the whole HPG Team, thank you for making my mission your mission. We are doing something very important, and you make it happen. None of this would be possible without my community of clients, both in-person and virtual, including my readers and everyone who joins me online for our many inspirational ventures. I love how savvy you have become and the way you bring that knowledge to every new person who comes into the fold. You are the reason I do what I do, and making your lives better makes my life better. Thank you for that.

Thank you to the amazing team that brought all of these food images to life! Aline Ponce and Michael Hulswit, Joe Lazo, Beryl Cohen, Jameson S. Pabes, Bayardo Ortiz, Katie Beth Umlor, you helped to make our photos gorgeous and special.

Finally, thank you to my crazy beautiful family: My parents, my sisters and sister in-law, my outlaw brothers, my cherished nieces and nephews, my outrageously precious kids, and my husband, who is the most handsome man in all the land! I love you with all my heart. Always have and always will! Now let's eat.

Haylie Pomroy

Index

Note: Page numbers in *italics* indicate illustrations.

Also by *New York Times* bestselling author

HAYLIE POMROY

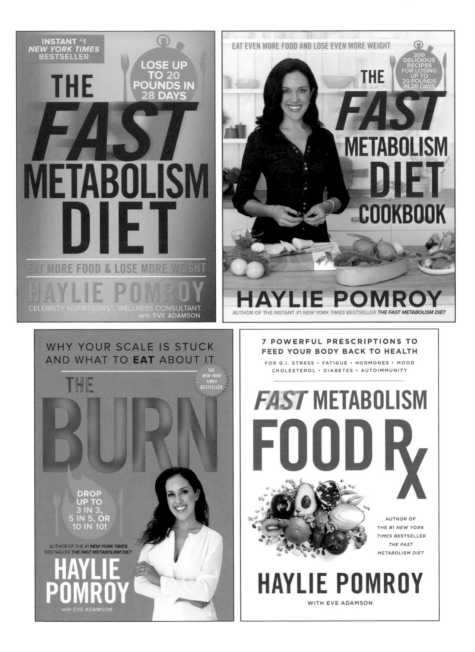

HARMONY

Available wherever books are sold